Windermere Ward ci

Practical Psoriasis Therapy

PRACTICAL PSORIASIS THERAPY

NICHOLAS J. LOWE, M.D., F.R.C.P., F.A.C.P.

Professor of Medicine/Dermatology
Director of Skin Disease
Psoriasis Treatment Center
UCLA School of Medicine
Los Angeles, California

YEAR BOOK MEDICAL PUBLISHERS, INC.
CHICAGO

0 9 8 7 6 5 4 3 2 1

Library of Congress Cataloging-in-Publication Data

Lowe, N. J. (Nicholas, J.)
  Practical psoriasis therapy.

  Includes bibliographies and index.
    1. Psoriasis—Treatment. I. Title. [DNLM: 1. Pso-
riasis—therapy. WR 205 L913p]
RL321.L69 1986   616.5'2606   85-17965
ISBN 0-8151-5642-1

Sponsoring editor: Susan M. Harter/David K. Marshall
Manager, copyediting services: Frances M. Perveiler
Production project manager: Sharon W. Pepping
Proofroom supervisor: Shirley E. Taylor

Contributors

THOMAS F. ANDERSON, M.D.
Associate Professor of Dermatology, Department of Dermatology, University of Michigan, Ann Arbor, Michigan

BRIAN S. ANDREWS, M.B., M.D., F.R.A.C.P., F.A.C.P.
Associate Professor of Medicine, Division of Rheumatology, Clinical Immunology, University of California, Irvine, Irvine, California

RICHARD E. ASHTON, M.B., M.R.C.P.
Consultant in Dermatology, Royal Navy Hospital Haslar, Gospost, Hampshire, England

MARC D. CHALET, M.D.
Adjunct Assistant Professor, Medicine/Dermatology, Director of Dermatopathology, UCLA School of Medicine, Los Angeles, California

ROGER C. CORNELL, M.D.
Chief, Division of Dermatology, Scripps Clinic, Memorial Group, Inc., LaJolla, California

MARY E. HARTMAN, M.D.
Resident, Department of Dermatology, University of California, Irvine, Irvine, California

STEPHEN HORWITZ, M.D.
Director of Phototherapy, Department of Dermatology, Mt. Sinai Medical Center, Miami Beach, Florida

T.P. KINGSTON, M.B., M.R.C.P.
Visiting Instructor, Division of Dermatology, UCLA School of Medicine, Los Angeles, California

NICHOLAS J. LOWE, M.D., F.R.C.P., F.A.C.P.
Professor of Medicine/Dermatology, Director of Skin Disease, and Psoriasis Treatment Center, UCLA School of Medicine, Los Angeles, California

M. ALAN MENTER, M.D.
Director, Psoriasis Treatment Center, Baylor College of Medicine, Dallas, Texas

RONALD L. MOY, M.D.
Chief Resident, Division of Dermatology, UCLA School of Medicine, Los Angeles, California

GERALD D. WEINSTEIN, M.D.
Professor and Chairman, Department of Dermatology, California College of Medicine, University of California, Irvine, Irvine, California

Preface

PSORIASIS remains a common disease of unknown etiology. While the etiology remains obscure, many new facts about the disease have been unearthed over the last two decades. This includes the knowledge that psoriasis appears to be an epidermal proliferative disorder. Also, there appears to be a significant inflammatory response within the skin. Although there is some evidence that a defect in epidermal differentiation may exist, it is not known if this is secondary to the inflammatory and epidermal proliferative components.

Most currently available and investigative treatments for this disease may work by a variety of mechanisms. The purpose of this book is not to review in detail the current theories on pathogenesis of the disease nor the mechanisms of possible actions of the different forms of therapy. Rather, the major purpose of *Practical Psoriasis Therapy* is to provide clinicians with a concise yet comprehensive reference about the important therapies that are now available and that may become available in the near future for the management of this chronic and relapsing skin problem. In addition to providing necessary background about the different forms of therapy, the authors have also attempted to give practical guidelines to facilitate implementation of suggested forms of therapy by physicians and to provide information for patients that may help improve their compliance.

Practical Psoriasis Therapy is intended for a broader audience than just dermatologists because in many instances, both here and abroad, the initial management of psoriasis falls to primary care physicians, including family physicians, internists, and pediatricians. In addition, rheumatologists treating psoriatic arthritis patients may be questioned about the different forms of therapy available for the treatment of the skin psoriasis problem. It is hoped, therefore, that *Practical Psoriasis Therapy* will provide the reader with some new and practical insights about different forms of psoriasis therapy, as well as with some proven and personal concepts of psoriasis therapy from a group of physicians who frequently treat patients with this disease.

Finally, I wish to bring to the attention of the reader some information and instructive literature for patients that I have found useful to help the patient understand and remember information discussed during consultation.

The editor would like to thank and acknowledge the support of American Dermal Corporation, Elder Pharmaceuticals, Glaxo Laboratories, Hoffmann-La Roche, Inc., Neutrogena Corporation, Ortho Pharmaceutical Corporation, Owen Laboratories, Westwood Pharmaceuticals, Inc., and The Skin and Research Foundation of California to enable the publishing of the color illustrations in this book.

NICHOLAS J. LOWE, M.D., F.R.C.P., F.A.C.P.

Foreword

PRACTICAL PSORIASIS THERAPY has been written as a practical guide and review of the most currently used therapies for psoriasis.

Psoriasis remains a difficult and puzzling disease, and there is a wide variety of different treatments available. These treatments have to be selected with great care based on the physician's experience as well as the patient's previous experiences and history.

Dr. Lowe has selected the most important therapies and both general and practical information about their usage. The book has been written as a guide for physicians who are required to manage this difficult disease.

Dr. Lowe is ideally suited to be editor of this book because he has been actively involved in the research and therapy of psoriasis for many years.

The contributors of this book are also involved in active clinical practice and research of different aspects of the disease and its therapy. They all have valuable insight and experience in managing patients with this disease. They were given the task of writing about the background and important practical aspects of different forms of therapy.

The introductory chapter presents an algorithm for the selection of psoriasis therapy. This will be useful in making the therapeutic choices for different patients. It provides a logical introduction to the later chapters.

The book is directed mainly toward the dermatologist, but other physicians including internists, rheumatologists, pediatricians, and family practitioners will find this book of great value when taking care of psoriasis patients. Practical aspects are stressed throughout with some helpful patient instructions that may be used as a basis for therapy and care.

JOHN J. VOORHEES, M.D.
PROFESSOR AND CHAIRMAN
DEPARTMENT OF DERMATOLOGY
UNIVERSITY OF MICHIGAN MEDICAL CENTER
ANN ARBOR, MICHIGAN

Contents

COLOR PLATES

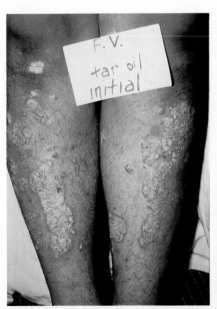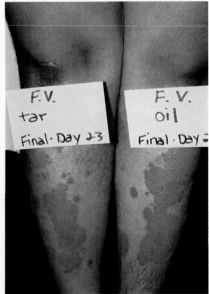

Plate 1.—Clinical photographs of the legs of a patient with plaques of chronic psoriasis vulgaris. **Left,** pretreatment. **Right,** 23 days after once-daily tar oil treatment to one leg and oil without tar to the other leg. Both legs are improved, but tar-treated leg shows more improvement than leg treated with oil only. No phototherapy was used. (From Lowe N.J., et al.: Coal tar phototherapy for psoriasis re-evaluated. *J. Amer. Acad. Dermatol.* 8:781–789, 1983. Reproduced by permission.)

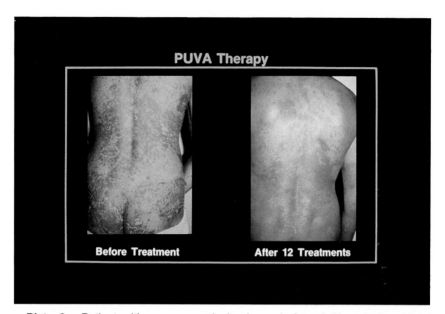

Plate 2.—Patient with severe psoriasis shown before *(left)* and after *(right)* oral methoxysalen and ultraviolet-A radiation (PUVA) therapy. (From Lowe N.J.: Psoriasis: The Disease and its Treatment. Herbert Laboratories, Irvine, California, 1983. Reproduced by permission.)

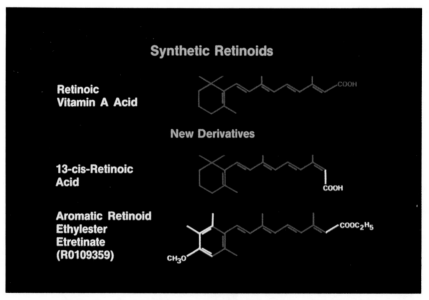

Plate 3.—Three different synthetic retinoids in clinical use.

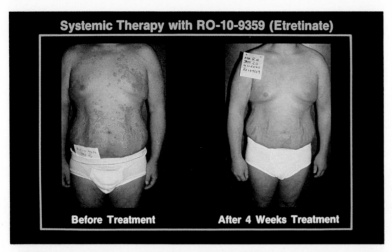

Systemic Therapy with RO-10-9359 (Etretinate)

Before Treatment   **After 4 Weeks Treatment**

Plate 4.—Results of treatment with etretinate. *Left,* before treatment; *right,* after treatment. (From Lowe N.J.: Psoriasis: The Disease and its Treatment. Herbert Laboratories, Irvine, California, 1983. Reproduced by permission.)

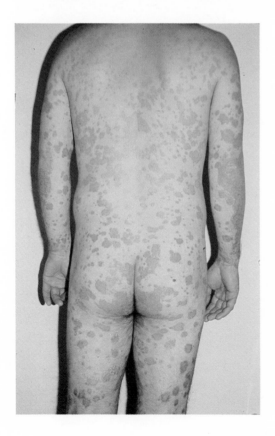

Plate 5.—Patient with extensive guttate psoriasis.

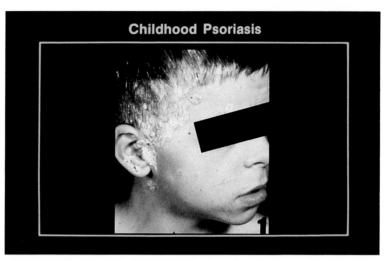

Plate 6.—Patient with severe scalp psoriasis. (From Lowe N.J.: Psoriasis: The Disease and its Treatment. Herbert Laboratories, Irvine, California, 1983. Reproduced by permission.)

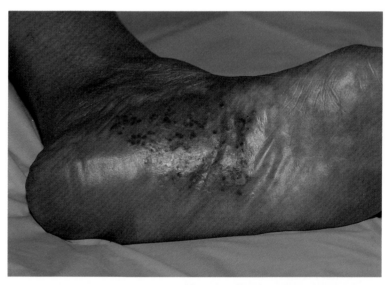

Plate 7.—Localized pustular psoriasis. More localized pustular forms of psoriasis usually occur on the palms and soles and may also be termed "pustular psoriasis of the palms and soles" or "pustular bacterid of Andrews." It may also be described as "acrodermatitis continua of Hallopeau," particularly when there is extensive digital involvement and periungual involvement with resultant finger and toe deformity.

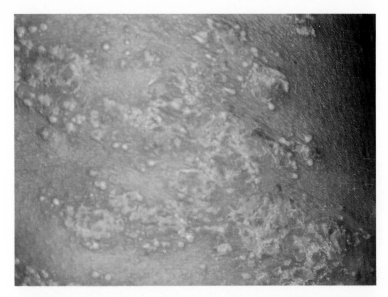

Plate 8.—Generalized pustular psoriasis. Yet another distinct clinical type is generalized pustular psoriasis. When the pustular psoriasis is generalized it may be accompanied by fever and malaise; this condition may be termed "generalized pustular psoriasis of Von Zumbusch."

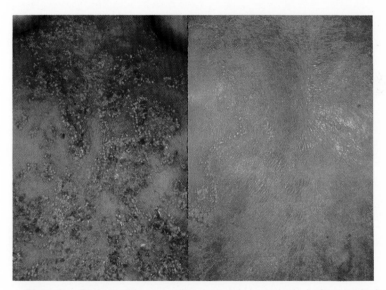

Plate 9.—Patient with generalized pustular psoriasis before and after 3 days treatment with oral 13-cis-retinoic acid. (From Sofen H., Moy R., Lowe N.J.: Treatment of generalized pustular psoriasis with isotretinoin. *Lancet* 40, Vol. 7, January 7, 1984. Reproduced by permission.)

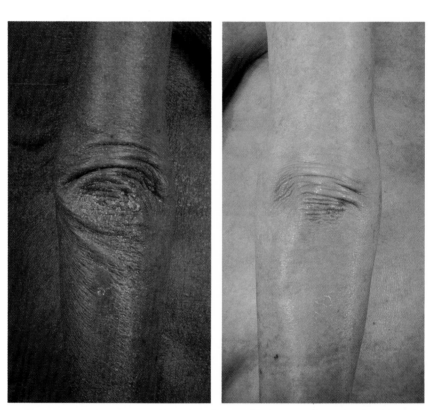

Plate 10.—**Left,** patient with exfoliative psoriasis remaining after four months of oral 13-cis-retinoic acid therapy. **Right,** same patient after six weeks of oral etretinate therapy.

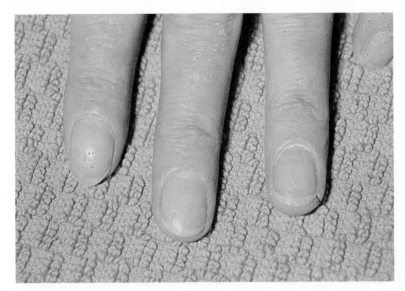

Plate 11.—Mild nail psoriasis, showing pitting of the nails. (From Lowe N.J.: Psoriasis: The Disease and its Treatment. Herbert Laboratories, Irvine, California, 1983. Reproduced by permission.)

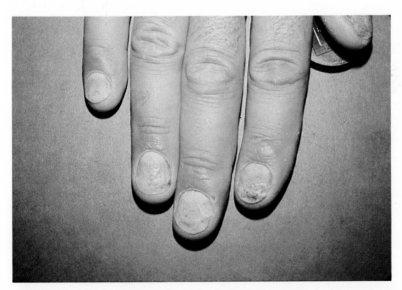

Plate 12.—More severe nail psoriasis than that shown in Plate 11, with onycholysis in addition to pitting. (From Lowe N.J.: Psoriasis: The Disease and its Treatment. Herbert Laboratories, Irvine, California, 1983. Reproduced by permission.)

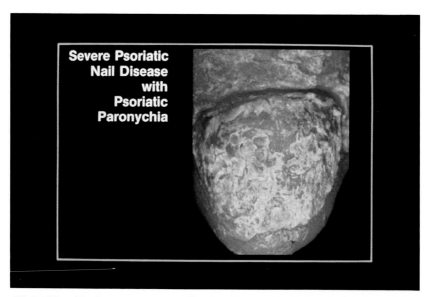

Plate 13.—Much more severe nail psoriasis than in two previous plates. Note marked nail dystrophy and hyperkeratosis. (From Lowe N.J.: Psoriasis: The Disease and its Treatment. Herbert Laboratories, Irvine, California, 1983. Reproduced by permission.)

1 / The Differential Diagnosis of Psoriasis

Nicholas J. Lowe, M.D., F.R.C.P., F.A.C.P.

THE DIAGNOSIS of classical untreated psoriasis on extensor skin surfaces usually presents no diagnostic problem for the dermatologist. However, psoriasis can be greatly modified by therapy which can make accurate clinical and histopathologic diagnosis difficult. In addition, the early stages of evolution of psoriasis can present the clinician with a diagnostic dilemma that is sometimes only resolved by the passage of time and the appearance of typical areas of clinical psoriasis and typical histopathologic changes on subsequent skin biopsy.

The importance of the accurate diagnosis of psoriasis is relevent to this book on psoriasis therapy. The relevance is the importance of knowing the patient has psoriasis because certain therapies are less appropriate for psoriasis than for other inflammatory dermatoses. As an example, systemic corticosteroids are often valuable in the management of certain forms of eczema but can be hazardous in the management of some patients with psoriasis.

This brief introductory chapter calls attention to many diseases that are commonly or less commonly confused with psoriasis.

The subsequent lists (Tables 1–1 through 1–8) were developed to highlight the differential diagnosis of different clinical types of psoriasis, with the differential diagnosis listed against each clinical type of psoriasis in the approximate order of frequency of presentation in the dermatology clinic. With these lists in mind, the reader is reminded that the classic onset of psoriasis is usually that of the plaque or guttate type of the disease.

In the *plaque* stage of the disease, the plaques are usually raised, erythematous patches with a classic silvery surface scale. If the scale is not apparent it usually can be made visible by gentle stroking or scratching of the psoriasis. The Auspitz sign (gentle lifting of the surface scale results in

1

TABLE 1–1.—Differential Diagnosis
of Psoriasis: Plaque Psoriasis Vulgaris

Frequent ↓ Less Frequent	Nummular Eczema
	Neurodermatitis
	Tinea Corporis
	Lichen Planus
	Lupus Erythematosus
	Benign Parapsoriasis
	Mycosis Fungoides
	Bowen's Squamous Carcinoma
	Hyperkeratotic Basal Cell Carcinoma
	Acrodermatitis Enteropathica (children)
	Pityriasis Rubra Pilaris (localized types)
	Zinc Deficiency

TABLE 1–2.—Differential Diagnosis
of Psoriasis: Flexural Psoriasis

Frequent ↓ Less Frequent	Seborrheic Eczema
	Diaper Dermatitis (children)
	Tinea Cruris
	Candidiasis
	Histiocytosis X (children)
	Perineal Bowen's Carcinoma
	Acrodermatis Enteropathica (children)

TABLE 1–3.—Differential
Diagnosis of Psoriasis:
Guttate Psoriasis

Frequent ↓ Less Frequent	Pityriasis Rosea
	Nummular Eczema
	Drug Eruptions
	Secondary Syphilis
	Benign Parapsoriasis
	Cutaneous Lymphoma

punctate bleeding from the prominent dermal capillaries) may be another helpful feature.

Guttate psoriasis is most commonly confused with pityriasis rosea; however, the lesions of guttate psoriasis are usually less oval than those of pityriasis rosea. There is usually more scale present in guttate psoriasis and the patient with guttate psoriasis is usually a child or teenager who gives a history of a significant upper respiratory tract infection, which is usually β-hemolytic streptococcal induced. This symptom can be confusing with pityriasis rosea because there may be feelings of malaise and upper respiratory infection prior to the onset of the pityriasis rosea.

TABLE 1–4.—DIFFERENTIAL DIAGNOSIS OF PSORIASIS: EXFOLIATIVE PSORIASIS

Frequent	Eczema: Atopic Dermatitis
	Seborrheic Dermatitis
	Other "Endogenous" Eczemas
	Contact Allergic Eczemas
	Drug Eruptions
	Idiopathic
	Pityriasis Rubra Pilaris
	Pityriasis Rosea
	Photosensitivity Skin Diseases
	Cutaneous Lymphomas
	Systemic Lymphomas
	Internal Malignancy
	Toxic Epidermal Necrolysis
	Lichen Planus
	Pemphigus
Less Frequent	Ichthyosiform Erythrodermas

TABLE 1–5.—DIFFERENTIAL DIAGNOSIS OF PSORIASIS: NAIL PSORIASIS

Frequent	Tinea Unguium
	Candidiasis
	Trauma
	Exfoliative Dermatitis (see list)
	Alopecia Areata
	Lichen Planus
	Drug-induced Onycholysis
	Twenty-nail Dystrophy
Less Frequent	Darier's Disease

TABLE 1–6.—DIFFERENTIAL DIAGNOSIS OF PSORIASIS: SCALP PSORIASIS

Frequent	Seborrheic Eczema
	Tinea Capitis
	Exfoliative Dermatitis (see list)
	Pityriasis Amiantacea
	Lupus Erythematosus
	Bowen's Carcinoma
	Drug Eruptions
Less Frequent	Pityriasis Rubra Pilaris

TABLE 1–7.—DIFFERENTIAL DIAGNOSIS OF PSORIASIS: PALMAR-PLANTAR PSORIASIS

Frequent	Eczema: Endogenous
	Contact Allergic
	Tinea Manum and Pedis
	Reiter's Syndrome
	Secondary Syphilis
	Scabies (children)
	Cutaneous Lymphoma
Less Frequent	Acrodermatitis Enteropathica (children)

TABLE 1–8.—Differential
Diagnosis of Psoriasis:
Generalized Pustular
Psoriasis (GPP)

Impetigo Herpetiformis in Pregnancy
  (probably variant of GPP)
Subcorneal Pustular Dermatosis
Pustular Drug Eruptions
Acrodermatitis Enteropathica (children)
Hypocalcemia

Other forms of psoriasis may be more subtle and confusing in their onset and frequently require the diagnostic skills of an experienced dermatologist for differentiation. Patients with pityriasis rubra pilaris, for example, have been referred to the author carrying a diagnosis of psoriasis. This is a problem because some of the therapies used for the treatment of psoriasis unfortunately exacerbate pityriasis rubra pilaris. Phototherapy worsens pityriasis rubra pilaris but usually helps psoriasis. It is therefore extremely valuable, as with all diseases, to obtain a complete and clear history as well as personal history, family history, and history of previous response to therapy.

An important differential diagnosis of scalp and flexural psoriasis is seborrheic eczema. Usually these patients have less thick scale and frequently facial involvement.

It should be remembered that psoriasis may coexist with other skin diseases and therapy may have to be appropriately modified.

The reader is also referred to Chapter 2, concerning the histopathology of psoriasis. Again, the reason for including this chapter in this text on psoriasis therapy is the vital importance of reaching a firm diagnosis of the disease prior to embarking on therapy.

2 / Histopathology of Psoriasis

MARC D. CHALET, M.D.

PSORIASIS IS A pathologic process that alters the appearance of the epidermis by increasing its thickness. The thickening of the epidermis may be accomplished in several ways. There may be an increase in the number of cells (hyperplasia), as seen in psoriasis, or an increase in individual cell size (hypertrophy), as seen in lichen simplex chronicus or lichen planus.

Hyperplasia occurs in four basic patterns, and combinations of these may occasionally be seen:

1. Irregular hyperplasia: uneven, elongated rete ridges with loss of the usual rete papillae configuration.

2. Papillated hyperplasia: digitate projections above the skin surface.

3. Pseudoepitheliomatous hyperplasia: massive elongation and distortion of the rete pattern to such a degree that it resembles a squamous cell carcinoma.

4. Psoriasiform hyperplasia: evenly elongated rete ridges with preservation and even accentuation of the rete papillae pattern. Psoriasis and the psoriasiform dermatitides display this fourth pattern of epidermal hyperplasia.[1]

In psoriasis, not only is the number of cells present within the epidermis increased, but the rate of epidermal cell proliferation is greatly accelerated. This acceleration includes a decrease in the transit time necessary for cells to move from the basal cell layer to the stratum corneum, as well as a decrease in the cell division cycle time.[6]

Electron microscopic studies have shown that keratinocytes within the regions where proliferation rates are increased (i.e., the psoriatic lesions) show significant abnormalities. These abnormalities include tonofilaments that are small and abnormally aggregated and a reduction in the size and number of keratohyaline granules present.[7] These electron microscopic changes indicate that the keratinocytes themselves are defective in psoriasis.

5

TABLE 2–1.—HISTOPATHOLOGIC EVOLUTION OF THE PSORIATIC LESION

	MACULES	SMALL PAPULES	LARGE SCALY PAPULES	LARGE PLAQUES	PUSTULES	RESOLVING LESIONS
Dilated and tortuous papillary dermal blood vessels	+	+	+ +	+ +	+ +	+
Papillary dermal edema	+	+ +	+ +	+ +	+ +	+
Superficial perivascular lymphocytic infiltrate	+	+ +	−	−	−	−
Spongiosis in epidermis	−	+	−	−	−	−
Superficial perivascular mixed-cell infiltrate with neutrophils	−	+	+ +	+ +	+ +	−
Superficial perivascular lymphohistiocytic infiltrate with siderophages and melanophages	−	−	−	−	−	+ +
Extravasated erythrocytes	+	− / +	+	+ +	− / +	−
Basket-weave stratum corneum	+	−	−	−	+	−
Compact orthokeratotic stratum corneum	−	+	+	−	− / +	+
Mitotic figures	−	+	+ +	+ +	− / +	−
Focal parakeratosis with neutrophils in stratum corneum	−	−	+ +	+	− / +	−
Confluent parakeratosis in stratum corneum	−	−	−	+ +	− / +	−
Psoriasiform hyperplasia of epidermis	− / +	+	+	+ +	− / +	− / +
Thin suprapapillary plates	−	−	−	+ +	− / +	+
Hypogranulosis	−	−	+	+ +	− / +	−
Pallid keratinocytes	−	−	+	+ +	− / +	−
Munro microabscesses	−	−	− / +	+	+	−
Spongioform pustules of Kogoj	−	−	− / +	+	+ +	−
Papillary dermal fibrosis	−	−	−	−	−	+

Key: − = absent; − / + = variable; + = present; + + = prominent.

The light microscopic features of psoriasis vary considerably with the age and type of lesion chosen for biopsy (Table 2–1). Some typical histologic features are illustrated in Figures 2–1 and 2–2.

The earliest and most persistent histologic sign of psoriasis is an increased tortuosity of the blood vessels in the dermal papillae. In early lesions, the vessels are surrounded by an infiltrate composed of scattered neutrophils and occasional extravasated erythrocytes. In older lesions, the infiltrate around these vessels and the vessels of the superficial papillary plexus is sparse and predominantly lymphohistiocytic. As the lesions continue to develop there is more prominent papillary dermal edema surrounding the dilated blood vessels. In the earliest macular lesions of psoriasis the changes are limited to the capillaries and venules of the superficial plexus.[2, 3] The inflammatory cell infiltrate around the superficial papillary plexus is sparse and lymphohistiocytic. The overlying epidermis and stratum corneum usually appear normal at this stage.

As the lesions progress to the early papular stage there is increased edema within the papillary dermis. Around the vessels of the superficial papillary plexus there is an inflammatory cell infiltrate composed predom-

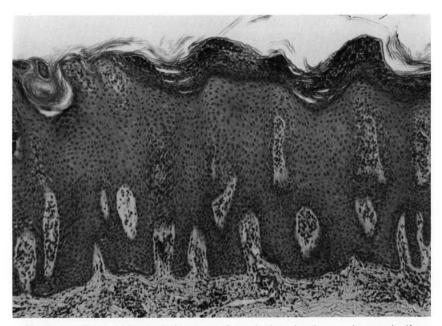

Fig 2–1.—Typical histologic features of psoriasis vulgaris: regular psoriasiform hyperplasia; dilated and tortuous blood vessels in the dermal papillae; thinned suprapapillary plates; diminished granular cell layer; confluent parakeratosis; and collections of neutrophils in stratum corneum ($\times 40$).

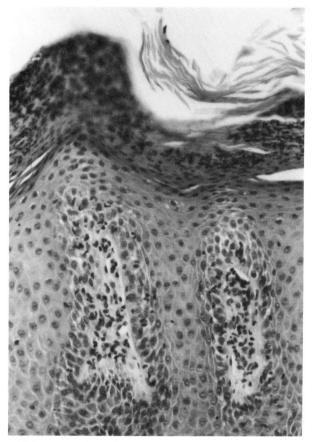

Fig 2–2.—High-power view of psoriasis vulgaris shows the same features as are seen in Fig 2–1, as well as mitoses in basal keratinocytes and collections of neutrophils in stratum corneum.

inantly of lymphocytes and histiocytes, as well as scattered neutrophils.[3] In the lower portions of the epidermis scattered mitotic figures can be seen within the keratinocytes and occasional foci of spongiosis are present. At this stage, some minimal hyperplasia of the epidermis may be noted. The overlying stratum corneum, which previously had a basket-weave appearance, now shows a focal compact orthokeratotic pattern. As the lesions progress further, all the features thus far described become more pronounced and there is a greater number of mitoses in the lower half of the epidermis.[5] Psoriasiform hyperplasia is slightly more prominent and zones of hypogranulosis can be seen in the granular layer.[4] In the overlying stratum corneum, parakeratosis is present above the hypogranulotic areas.

There are occasional neutrophils within the epidermis and small collections of neutrophils are present in the stratum corneum in association with the areas of parakeratosis.

If a biopsy is taken from a fully developed, large, scaly plaque of psoriasis, the changes present include a moderately dense, superficial, perivascular, lymphohistiocytic infiltrate containing scattered neutrophils, prominent edema of the papillary dermis, dilated and tortuous blood vessels within the dermal papillae, scattered, extravasated erythrocytes in the papillary dermis and occasionally within the epidermis, and marked psoriasiform hyperplasia with long, thin rete ridges that are equal in length.[1, 2] Occasionally the bases of the rete ridges are clubbed and fused with adjacent rete ridges. The portion of the epidermis above the dermal papillae (suprapapillary plates) is thinned, and the blood vessels within the dermal papillae are close to the stratum corneum. It is these last two features which account for the pinpoint bleeding that occurs if overlying scale is removed (the Auspitz sign). In the upper portion of the epidermis there is marked pallor of the keratinocytes resulting from intracellular edema.[2] Scattered spongioform pustules of Kogoj may be present within the epidermis, extending up to the stratum corneum. These spongioform pustules are aggregates of neutrophils and along with Munro microabscesses are distinctive in psoriatic lesions. The Munro microabscess is a collection of neutrophils mixed with the mounds of parakeratotic stratum corneum. In fully developed lesions of psoriasis the granular layer is almost completely absent and the stratum corneum demonstrates areas of confluent parakeratosis containing scattered neutrophils. These areas may be interspersed with foci of compact orthokeratosis.

If the psoriatic process is exaggerated, larger spongioform pustules, which may be termed macroabscesses, will be formed. This change is seen in pustular psoriasis. If this process is developing rapidly the large spongioform pustules will be formed before the epidermis has become hyperplastic. Spongioform pustules, therefore, may be seen without associated hyperplasia of the epidermis, especially in rapidly developing lesions.[1]

As lesions of psoriasis begin to regress, the feature which appeared last will be the first to disappear. The parakeratotic stratum corneum reverts to a compact orthokeratotic appearance. The granular layer begins to redevelop, most prominently in the center of the rete ridges. Psoriasiform hyperplasia becomes less prominent and the number of mitoses in evidence decreases. The suprapapillary plates may remain thinned. Still-prominent will be the dilated capillaries in the papillary dermis.[1, 2] As the papillary dermal edema recedes, there may be a slight increase in the number of fibroblasts present. Around the vessels of the superficial papillary plexus an infiltrate composed of lymphocytes, histiocytes, siderophages, and melanophages will be present.

REFERENCES

1. Ackerman A.B.: *Histopathologic Diagnosis of Inflammatory Skin Diseases.* Philadelphia, Lea & Febiger, 1978, pp. 250–256.
2. Ackerman A.B., Ragaz A.: *The Lives of Lesions.* New York, Masson Publishing, USA Inc., 1984, pp. 181–191.
3. Ragaz A., Ackerman A.B.: Evolution, maturation, and regression of lesions of psoriasis. *Am. J. Dermatopathol.* 1:199–214, 1979.
4. Soltani K., Van Scott E.J.: Patterns and sequence of tissue changes in incipient and evolving lesions of psoriasis. *Arch. Dermatol.* 106:484–490, 1972.
5. Van Scott E.J., Ekel T.W.: Kinetics of hyperplasia in psoriasis. *Arch. Dermatol.* 88:373–381, 1963.
6. Weinstein G.D., Frost P.: Abnormal cell proliferation in psoriasis. *J. Invest. Dermatol.* 50:254–259, 1968.
7. Walter F.L., Schaumburg-Lever G.: *Histopathology of the Skin*, ed. 6. Philadelphia, J.P. Lippincott, 1983, pp. 139–148.

3 / The Psoriasis Patient: Selection of Therapy

T. P. KINGSTON, M.B., M.R.C.P.
NICHOLAS J. LOWE, M.D., F.R.C.P., F.A.C.P.

WHEN A SINGLE disease has multiple alternative modes of therapy it is obvious that its etiology is unknown and that no one form of therapy is ideal. This is especially true of psoriasis, for which multiple alternative treatments have been used and are currently in use (Table 3–1). These many forms of therapy all have their benefits and drawbacks; no single treatment is ideal and it is rare for a patient not to be treated with several alternative treatments during his or her lifetime.

Many factors can influence the choice of therapy for psoriasis. It is a disease that can start at any age and run a relapsing and remitting course taking various clinical forms, e.g., chronic plaque, exfoliative, and generalized pustular. Usually the aim of treatment is to produce a clearing of the lesions, but we sometimes settle for the compromise of partial clearing

TABLE 3–1.—SOME
ALTERNATIVE FORMS OF
TREATMENT FOR PSORIASIS

1. Topical
Emollients and keratolytics
Tars
Anthralin
Topical steroids
   weak
   potent
2. Systemic
PUVA with oral psoralen
Methotrexate
Retinoids
3. Physical
UVB or topical psoralen plus UVA

11

Problem　　　　　　　　Possible Choices of Treatment　　　　　　Aim

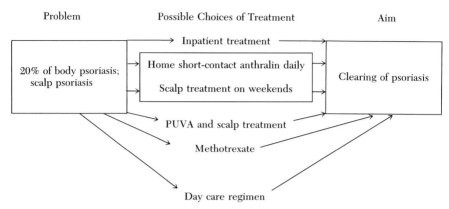

Fig 3–1.—Choosing a treatment regimen for the psoriasis patient described in the text. The form of treatment chosen depends on the type and extent of psoriasis as well as the patient's ability to comply with the requirements of therapy.

where a complete clearing and prolonged remission could only be achieved at the expense of unacceptable treatment toxicity.

The remainder of this chapter will attempt to highlight the difficulties experienced in choosing the correct form of psoriasis therapy and will give some introductory suggestions about the choice of therapy for different clinical circumstances.

Let us take, for example, a young man of 35 with family commitments who has psoriasis affecting 20% of his skin (Fig 3–1). He is unable to take time off work and he needs to be smartly dressed for his job, but he has a supportive family and time on weekends and nights that is available for home treatment. Inpatient therapy is not practical. Day-care treatment will take too much time from the day for this patient, requiring at least five hours daily. Psoralen with ultraviolet A (PUVA) and methotrexate are inappropriate at this stage because of potential side effects.

One practical solution is for him to use short-contact anthralin therapy at home in the evenings. He then showers the anthralin off the skin to avoid staining of his clothing and to reduce skin irritation. During weekdays he can shampoo his hair with a tar shampoo in the mornings and on the weekends he can use more messy and effective scalp treatments such as coal tar and salicylic acid in mineral oil, left on overnight and washed off in the morning. With this regimen it should be possible to achieve good improvement or clearing of his psoriasis within approximately six weeks. The treatments suggested here also give him a good chance of long remission of his disease.

Two major factors influencing choice of psoriasis therapy are the extent of the disease and the age of the patient (Table 3–2).

TABLE 3–2.—Major Factors
Influencing Choice
of Psoriasis Therapy

1. *Extent of Disease*
   a. Diffuse Guttate
   b. Localized small plaque
   c. Extensive large plaque
   d. Exfoliative
   e. Special sites
      (i) scalp
      (ii) flexures
      (iii) palms and soles
2. *Age of Patient*
   a. Child
   b. Healthy adult
   c. Elderly

The extent or type of the disease may be divided into the following subcategories.

Guttate psoriasis is often scattered and widespread with an abrupt onset and occasional spontaneous recovery in six weeks. Sometimes, however, it is more persistent and requires therapy. An ideal form of therapy for acute widespread guttate psoriasis is the use of purified tar and ultraviolet-B phototherapy.

Localized small-plaque psoriasis on the elbows and knees may be adequately treated with anthralin.

Extensive plaque psoriasis may require tar, anthralin, and ultraviolet-B phototherapy. In general, the more extensive the disease, the greater is the need for treatment at a specialized center. PUVA or systemic therapy may be required for some patients.

Exfoliative psoriasis usually requires treatment in a day-care center or hospital. Initial topical corticosteroids to reduce erythroderma, followed by Goeckerman or PUVA therapy, is a useful plan. Systemic therapy with a synthetic retinoid, such as etretinate or methotrexate, may be required.

Some body sites may require special treatment for psoriasis:

Scalp psoriasis usually requires a treatment to reduce scaling. Effective agents for this include coal tar and salicylic acid creams and ointments, as well as the cautious use of anthralin to the scalp.

Flexures often require milder-strength topical corticosteroids, plus antimycotic, antimicrobial agents. Flexural skin may be irritated by coal tar and usually requires a mild-potency steroid cream.

Palm and sole psoriasis is always difficult to treat topically, as topical agents are only partially successful, perhaps because of percutaneous pen-

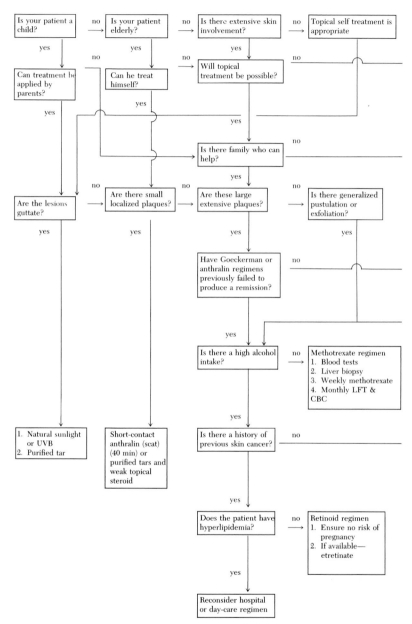

Fig 3–2.—Clinical algorithm for selecting psoriasis therapy.

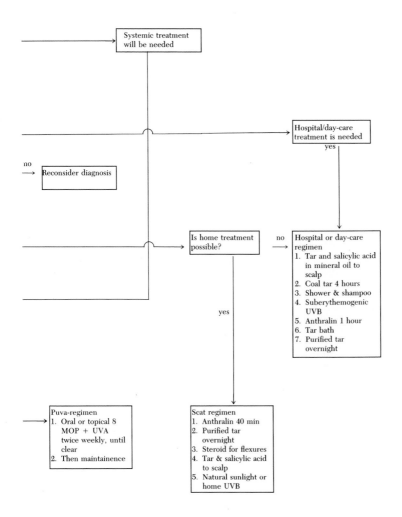

Systemic treatment will be needed

Hospital/day-care treatment is needed
yes

no
Reconsider diagnosis

Is home treatment possible?

no
Hospital or day-care regimen
1. Tar and salicylic acid in mineral oil to scalp
2. Coal tar 4 hours
3. Shower & shampoo
4. Suberythemogenic UVB
5. Anthralin 1 hour
6. Tar bath
7. Purified tar overnight

yes

Puva-regimen
1. Oral or topical 8 MOP + UVA twice weekly, until clear
2. Then maintainence

Scat regimen
1. Anthralin 40 min
2. Purified tar overnight
3. Steroid for flexures
4. Tar & salicylic acid to scalp
5. Natural sunlight or home UVB

etration problems in the area. PUVA phototherapy or systemic therapy may be required for this localized but often disabling form of psoriasis.

The patient's age may be divided into three categories.

A *child* will usually have topical therapy applied by the parents. Although the parents may worry greatly about the skin's appearance, the child may not. Compliance, therefore, will hinge on the ability of the parent to encourage the continued use of therapy. A fixed routine is necessary; for example, nightly treatment after bathtime. If there are difficulties with treatment applications it is often better to have treatment performed in a day-care center or hospital setting so that parents can be shown the correct way to apply ointments and creams and future effective treatment habits be established.

Healthy adults are, of course, responsible for their own treatment compliance; however, they may require help with the therapy, for example in treatment of the back skin and the scalp. Ideally the family can help, but again, day-care center or hospital treatment may be necessary.

Elderly patients usually need treatments to be applied for them, either because of relative immobility or lack of volition. In addition, some elderly people have different forms of arthritis and cannot apply treatments themselves. If home treatment cannot be performed with success then day care or inpatient hospital treatment will be necessary or the use of systemic therapy considered.

In deciding between topical or systemic therapy, always use topical therapy unless there is some overriding consideration—for example, previous failure of topical therapy, inability to apply topical therapy, rapid relapse after previous therapy, the presence of severe psoriatic arthritis, or such extensive disease that systemic therapy is appropriate.

SYSTEMIC TREATMENTS

When considering systemic therapy, one should have full knowledge of the available treatments and the ability to monitor the patient's progress. Appropriate screening tests for side effects are essential; for example, blood tests and liver biopsies should be performed before and during methotrexate therapy. There are obvious contraindications for each of the systemic treatments: for example, alcohol intake with methotrexate, hyperlipidemia or possibility of pregnancy with the retinoids, and previous skin cancers with PUVA.

PSORIASIS THERAPY ALGORITHM

The following algorithm (Fig 3–2) was constructed to illustrate the decision-making process for choosing the appropriate therapy for a patient's psoriasis. This is based on our personal preferences and aimed to produce a maximum improvement or clearance for the patient. We have assumed that all possible choices of treatment are available, although this may not be the case.

Frequently the cost of therapy is a major consideration, particularly to the patient without comprehensive health care insurance coverage in the United States and other countries.

One final suggestion is to allow both patient and physician sufficient time to consider the most appropriate form of therapy. Before embarking upon any form of treatment, the patient should understand what is expected in terms of compliance, as well as what he or she can expect as a result. Factors that should be taken into account—not necessarily in order of importance—include safety, efficacy, practicality, and cost.

The treatment regimen should then be followed until a clearing is achieved and not discarded before an adequate trial of therapy. This is particularly important with anthralin treatment and different types of phototherapy.

Psoriasis very rarely is a fatal disease, although severe disability often occurs. Some forms of therapy, however, do have significant risk of morbidity and occasional mortality and the correct choice of therapy is of critical importance in this skin disease. It is hoped that this chapter and the subsequent chapters of this book will assist in choosing the appropriate course of therapy for the psoriasis patient.

4 / Topical Steroids

ROGER C. CORNELL, M.D.

A MULTIPLICITY of topical steroids is available to the practitioner for the treatment of psoriasis. Such agents are available as ointments, creams, lotions, aerosols, and steroid-impregnated tape. In treating psoriasis the practitioner must consider the potency of the agent used, the frequency of application, the location of the lesion and the degree to which the lesion is steroid-sensitive or steroid-resistant. Psoriasis is considered to be both a steroid-sensitive and a steroid-resistant dermatosis. Thick, plaque-type psoriatic lesions on the elbows or the knees are considered steroid-resistant and require aggressive topical therapy, whereas psoriatic lesions on the penis, in the body folds, and on the scrotum tend to be less thickened and more erythematous and are considered steroid-sensitive. The palms and soles, for example, are extremely thick so that topical agents tend to penetrate these areas less well than areas where the skin is thin, such as the eyelids, body folds, and groin.

Topical glucocorticosteroids can be ranked into seven potency categories. Table 4–1 summarizes the potencies of the currently available topical glucocorticosteroids.

CHOOSING A STEROID

Topical steroids should be used as an adjunct to other accepted forms of topical therapy, such as tar derivatives, ultraviolet light, etc., but not exclusive of them. As noted earlier, the steroid to be selected to treat a psoriatic lesion is a function of the site of the lesion, the severity of the lesion, and the steroid's inherent potency.

18

TABLE 4-1.—CURRENTLY AVAILABLE TOPICAL GLUCOCORTICOSTEROIDS*

BRAND NAME	GENERIC NAME
Group I	
Diprolene ointment 0.5%†	Betamethasone dipropionate in optimized vehicle
Group II	
Cyclocort ointment 0.1%	Amcinonide
Diprosone ointment 0.05%	Betamethasone dipropionate
Florone ointment 0.05%	Diflorasone diacetate
Halog cream 0.1%	Halcinonide
Lidex cream 0.05%	Fluocinonide
Lidex ointment 0.05%	Fluocinonide
Maxiflor ointment 0.05%	Diflorasone diacetate
Topicort cream 0.25%	Desoximethasone
Topicort ointment 0.25%	Desoximethasone
Topsyn gel 0.05%	Fluocinonide
Group III	
Aristocort cream (HP) 0.5%	Triamcinolone acetonide
Diprosone cream 0.05%	Betamethasone dipropionate
Florone cream 0.05%	Diflorasone diacetate
Maxiflor cream 0.05%	Diflorasone diacetate
Valisone ointment 0.1%	Betamethasone valerate
Group IV	
Aristocort ointment 0.1%	Triamcinolone acetonide
Benisone ointment 0.025%	Betamethasone benzoate
Cordran ointment 0.05%	Flurandrenolide
Kenalog ointment 0.1%	Triamcinolone acetonide
Synalar cream (HP) 0.2%	Fluocinolone acetonide
Synalar ointment 0.025%	Fluocinolone acetonide
Topicort LP cream 0.05%	Desoximethasone
Group V	
Benisone cream 0.025%	Betamethasone benzoate
Cordran cream 0.05%	Flurandrenolide
Diprosone lotion 0.02%	Betamethasone dipropionate
Kenalog cream 0.1%	Triamcinolone acetonide
Kenalog lotion 0.1%	Triamcinolone acetonide
Locoid cream 0.1%	Hydrocortisone butyrate
Synalar cream 0.025%	Fluocinolone acetonide
Valisone cream 0.1%	Betamethasone valerate
Valisone lotion 0.1%	Betamethasone valerate
Westcort cream 0.2%	Hydrocortisone valerate
Group VI	
Tridesilon cream 0.05%	Desonide
Locorten cream 0.03%	Flumethasone pivalate
Synalar solution 0.01%	Fluocinolone acetonide
Group VII	
Topicals with hydrocortisone, dexamethasone, flumethalone, prednisolone and methylprednisolone	

*Groups are arranged in descending order of potency. There is no significant difference of agents within any given group; within each group the compounds are arranged alphabetically.

†Package insert calls for no more than 45 gm per week for two weeks followed by a rest period.

Scalp

Psoriatic lesions on the scalp may range from thick, ostraceous lesions to relatively mild erythema and scaling. In general, patients do not like to use ointments on the scalp and many patients will not use creams either. Steroids have been developed in lotion form and in gel form for use on the scalp. In addition, aerosol sprays with a nozzle adaptor are frequently helpful in enabling the steroid to be delivered to the scalp. Lotions, sprays, and gels can be rubbed into the scalp more easily than creams and ointments and are to be recommended in the treatment of scalp psoriasis.

Face

Because of the ability of topical steroids to cause atrophy, telangiectasia, rosacea, and acneiform eruptions, the use of potent steroids on the face is to be avoided. When psoriasis occurs on the face, it is usually mild and should be treated with a relatively weak steroid, such as one from Group VI or VII (see Table 4–1). If the lesions on the face are dry and fissured, then an ointment base can be used; otherwise, a cream base can be utilized. In general, most patients find aerosols on the nonhairy areas of the body overly drying.

Trunk

The type of psoriatic lesions present on the trunk varies from plaque-type to guttate-type and in some instances to pustular psoriasis. Ointments, creams, or gels may be used on the trunk areas. Most patients prefer to use creams on covered areas of the skin and their effectiveness may be enhanced by occlusion using plastic wrap. If a patient is willing to use an ointment on covered areas, by all means use it. Ointments are inherently more clinically effective than simple creams or lotions, since the ointment base tends to enhance penetration.

Extremities

Lesions on the extremities, particularly the lower extremities, are notoriously difficult to treat. Psoriatic lesions in these areas often are plaque-type and quite thick. The use of a potent steroid in an ointment base or a steroid in a cream base under occlusion is often necessary, particularly for thick, ostraceous plaques. If a relatively small number of lesions is present, then a steroid-impregnated tape (Cordran tape) may be utilized. The tape should be applied 1–2 hours after bathing and left on for 12–16 hours. The steroid-impregnated tapes are expensive and thus should be reserved for small numbers of lesions or problem areas.

Palms and Soles

Topical steroids are only mildly effective in the treatment of psoriasis on the palms and soles. Even the most potent agents (Group I on Table 4–1) have not resulted in significant clinical improvement in psoriasis of the palms. If the patient is willing, a potent steroid cream under occlusion can be utilized. The mid- to lower-strength topical agents have relatively little effect on the treatment of psoriasis on the palms and soles.

Nail Folds

The use of topical steroids on nail folds is relatively unrewarding, probably because even the most potent agents are unable to penetrate adequately to the nail matrix area. The use of intralesional steroids on the proximal nail folds should be considered. The authors use a dilution of 4 mg of Kenalog per cc of Xylocaine. While the procedure is often effective, it is painful and does require the patient to be seen every 4–6 weeks for repeat injections as needed. Patients with twenty-nail disease might not be good candidates for repeat interlesional injections, but a psoriatic with only several nails involved might be considered a candidate for this form of therapy. In general, we use no more than 1–2 mg per proximal nail fold.

Body Folds

Psoriatic lesions in body folds tend to be primarily erythematous, with minimal scaling. One of the reasons for this may be that mechanical factors such as walking tends to move the hyperkeratotic debris. Since the lesions have less hyperkeratosis, steroids tend to penetrate better; in addition, since the skin in the body fold area tends to be thin, one should begin with a low potency steroid to areas such as the penis, the vaginal area, etc. In general, patients do not like ointments in these areas and creams or gels are often better accepted.

We recommend using no more than 45 gm weekly of a medium-strength to potent steroid in adult patients and no more than 15 gm of a mild-to-weak strength steroid in children. It is often difficult to get good patient compliance when the frequency of application is 3–4 times a day and quite likely application twice daily of most steroids will suffice. As noted above, the potency of the steroid should be no stronger than necessary to treat the dermatologic condition.

There are approximately 12 different 0.5% hydrocortisone products currently available over the counter. Over-the-counter hydrocortisone is to be recommended primarily for use in body fold areas where a weak topical agent will suffice.

TOPICAL SIDE EFFECTS

Multiple topical side effects have been described with the use of topical agents. The practitioner must be aware that these side effects increase as one increases the potency of the agent and as one uses the agent on areas of the body where the skin is inherently thin.

Striae and Atrophy

Usually this is not seen until an agent has been used for more than three weeks. When a potent agent is used the occurrence of striae and atrophy must be carefully monitored. If detected early, atrophy and striae are frequently reversible once the offending agent is discontinued. Thinning of the dermis and epidermis and prominent telangiectatic changes, may, however, be permanent.[1] The use of potent topical steroids in areas already thinned from the sun (extensor arm area, sides of the neck, etc.) or in body folds may result in purpuric changes and even in lacerations secondary to mild trauma, which may raise skin flaps and subcutaneous tissue from the deep fascia.

The development of striae and atrophy is a particular problem in infants and young children since the skin of patients in this age group is inherently thinner. Long-term application of all but the least potent steroids should be avoided in the pediatric patient.

Perioral Dermatitis

Perioral dermatitis is a common side effect resulting from the misuse of potent topical steroids on the face.[2] Treatment consists of discontinuation of the agent and administration of tetracycline at a dose of 250–500 mg per day for a 4–6-week period.

Acne

Plewig and Kligman[3] have reported the induction of an acneiform eruption in human adult male volunteers by the topical application of various commercial steroid creams. Fortunately, acne scarring following steroidal-induced acne is unusual, possibly due to the agents' anti-inflammatory capabilities.

Rosacea

The term *steroid rosacea*[4] has been used to describe the development of a combination of erythema, telangiectasia and atrophy together with papules and pustules on the face in patients who have received mid-strength to potent steroids for minor facial eruptions. Treatment consists of discontinuation of the steroid; the use of tetracycline may also be required in a low-dose schedule.

Glaucoma

Virtually all topical steroids can result in glaucoma when used about the eyes.[5, 6] All but the weakest steroids should be avoided around the eyes and the patient should use even weak agents only on a limited basis in this area.

Secondary Infection

Whether topical steroids cause tinea infections is poorly understood. Suffice it to say that topical steroids, particularly in an ointment form, may produce enough occlusion and maceration that a secondary tinea infection is able to occur. In addition, topical steroids may mask another process, such as tinea, by reducing inflammation of the diseased skin.[7]

Allergic Contact Dermatitis

This has been reported with some steroids.[8] In most instances, it is not the steroid itself but the vehicle the agent is mixed with that is the culprit.

SYSTEMIC SIDE EFFECTS

If enough steroid is used over a large enough area, particularly under occlusion, to diseased skin, suppression of the pituitary-adrenal axis may occur. This has been reported even with steroids of mild potency.[9] The practitioner must be particularly aware of pituitary-adrenal axis suppression when he uses one of the most potent steroids. Application of 0.1% halcinonide cream to subjects with psoriasis was shown to cause a decrease of plasma cortisol on the mornings after treatment over a 5-day period when 15 gm was applied to approximately 50% of the body daily without occlusion.[10]

Nine out of 22 patients treated with 0.25% desoximethasone emollient cream daily for six months had a transient fall of plasma cortisol levels during the treatment period. An average of 9.8 gm was used daily to psoriatic skin without occlusion.[11] Betamethasone dipropionate ointment in a new optimized vehicle (diprolene) may cause suppression of the pituitary-adrenal axis if more than 45 gm is used weekly. The package insert calls for use of no more than 45 gm weekly for two weeks, followed by a rest period.

In Britain, clobetasol propionase 0.05% cream and ointment has been used for many years. As little as 30 gm of this compound in the ointment base applied to normal skin daily for 4½ days has been reported to suppress the pituitary-adrenal axis. When patients with diseased skin covering 5%–50% of the body surface used over 50 gm weekly, the plasma cortisol levels consistently fell to below normal limits.[12]

Cushing's syndrome fortunately is rare but can occur, particularly when the topical agent is flagrantly misused. Thirty grams daily of desoximethasone emollient cream 0.25% on psoriatic skin, for example, has been reported to cause florid Cushing's syndrome and hirsutism.[13] As opposed to the endogenous form of Cushing's syndrome, in which the plasma cortisol is markedly elevated and cannot be suppressed, the plasma cortisol in iatrogenic Cushing's syndrome is decreased.

Unfortunately, there is as yet no topical steroid formulation available in this country whose clinical potency does not parallel both topical and systemic side effects.

ACTION OF STEROIDS

Topical steroids are believed to act in several ways in the treatment of psoriasis: (1) vasoconstriction—by inducing vasoconstriction steroids reduce erythema, a manifestation of psoriasis; (2) decreased cell turnover— by slowing cellular proliferation steroids are useful in treating cutaneous disorders marked by rapid cellular turnover, such as psoriasis; and (3) antiinflammatory action—because of their effects on leukocytes, topical steroids reduce inflammation and hence are useful in conditions such as psoriasis in which leukocytes may play a role. The site of activity of glucocorticoids in the skin is not known. It is likely that all cells have specific receptors for glucocorticoids.

A common observation in the treatment of psoriasis is that the patient may seem to develop resistance to the use of a topical agent in the treatment of his or her disease. This may be secondary to acute tolerance to the drug (tachyphylaxis).[14] If after four to six weeks the psoriatic lesion becomes resistant to the topical therapy, consideration of temporarily discontinuing the agent and the initiation of a different agent might be in order. The ability of potent steroids to cause a pustular flare of psoriasis means that the practitioner must use these agents cautiously, particularly when more than 45 gm per week is used. Clobetasol propionate has been reported to cause a pustular flare in several psoriatic patients treated with high doses.[15] When a pustular flare occurs, a patient may need to be weaned off the potent agent by using progressively weaker agents over a many-month time period. Systemic therapy may be required to control pustular flares.

The use of intralesional therapy may be of great benefit in the treatment of localized areas of psoriasis. Psoriatic lesions can be injected with Kenalog mixed with Xylocaine, 4 mg per cc. In general, injections should be reserved for only steroid-resistant areas of psoriasis. The authors rarely use more than a total dose of 8 mg of triamcinolone nor administer more than 2 mg for a 2 × 2 cm treatment site. Since measurable amounts of the steroid remain in the skin and are released for three to four weeks after treatment, injections should be given no more than every four to six weeks.

TABLE 4–2.—TOPICAL CORTICOSTEROID (STEROID) THERAPY
IN PSORIASIS: PATIENT INSTRUCTIONS

These are often very effective preparations, but they have to be used with care.
Only apply *small* amounts of them *twice daily* to psoriasis skin, unless advised otherwise by
your physician. Rub them well into your psoriasis.
Do not continue treating after the psoriasis has cleared; this can lead to skin thinning.
Do not apply any steroid to the *face* or skin folds unless specifically advised by your physician.
If any new skin irritation, skin bruising, ulcers, or skin infections occur, *stop* using the corti-
costeroid therapy until you have checked with your physician.

The ability of Kenalog mixed with Xylocaine to cause atrophy must be kept
in mind, particularly when lesions on the neck, face, or intergluteal areas
are injected.

PATIENT INSTRUCTIONS

Table 4–2 is a sample instruction sheet for patients using topical corticosteroids. In discussing the topical use of steroids with patients, we advise
them that most patients use far too much of the topical agent. The material
should be rubbed in gently. If, after rubbing the agent in, any cream remains visible on the surface skin, then more than the necessary amount
has been used. The patient should avoid applying the agent to areas of
healthy skin. This is somewhat difficult if the patient has multiple, small
guttate lesions over numerous areas of the body; even so, the patient
should avoid the use of the agent to normal skin to decrease the risk of
side effects. In addition, topical steroids are expensive. Patients should be
specifically advised only to use the agent on the area designated. Often the
patient feels that if an agent is good for one area of the body, it must be
good for other sites and conditions as well. Always indicate to the patient
the area to be treated and the frequency of application. Never write a
prescription for unlimited refills. When using the more potent topical
agents, the patient should be seen every two to three months to monitor
efficacy and potential side effects.

REFERENCES

1. Stevanovic D.V.: Corticosteroid-induced atrophy of the skin with telangiectasia. *Br. J.
Dermatol.* 87:548–556, 1972.
2. Sneddon I.: Perioral dermatitis. *Br. J. Dermatol.* 87:430–434, 1972.
3. Plewig G., Kligman A.M.: Induction of acne by topical steroids. *Arch. Dermatol. Forsch.*
247:29–51, 1973.

4. Leyden J.J., Thew M., Kligman A.M.: Steroid rosacea. *Arch. Dermatol.* 110:619–622, 1974.
5. Koss M.A., Kolker A.E., Becker B.: Chronic topical corticosteroid use stimulating congenital glaucoma. *J. Pediatr.* 81:1175–1177, 1972.
6. Castrow F.F.: Atopic cataracts versus steroid cataracts. *J. Am. Acad. Derm.* 5:64–66, 1981.
7. Ive F.A., Marks R.: Tinea incognito. *Br. Med. J.* 3:149–152, 1968.
8. Alani M.D., Alani S.D.: Allergic contact dermatitis to corticosteroids. *Ann. Allergy* 30:181–185, 1972.
9. Scoggins R.B., Kliman B.: Percutaneous absorption of corticosteroids. *N. Engl. J. Med.* 273:832–840, 1965.
10. Gomez E.C., Kaminester L., Frost P.: Topical halcinonide and betamethasone valerate effects on plasma cortisol. *Arch. Dermatol.* 113:1196–1202, 1977.
11. Cornell R., Stoughton R.B.: Six-month controlled study of effect of desoximetasone and betamethasone-17-valerate on the pituitary-adrenal axis. *Br. J. Dermatol.* 105:91–95, 1981.
12. Ortega E., Burdick K.H., Segre, E.J.: Adrenal suppression by clobetasol propionate. *Lancet* 1:1200, 1975.
13. Himathongkam T., Dasanabhairochana P., Pilchayayothin N.: Florid Cushing's syndrome and hirsutism by desoximetasone. *JAMA* 239:430–431, 1978.
14. du Vivier A., Stoughton R.B.: Tachyphylaxis to the action of topically applied corticosteroids. *Arch. Dermatol.* 111:581–583, 1975.
15. Carruthers J.A., August P.J., Staughton R.C.D.: Observations on the systemic effect of topical clobetasol propionate (Dermovate). *Br. Med. J.* 4:203–204, 1975.

5 / Tars, Keratolytics and Emollients

Nicholas J. Lowe, M.D., F.R.C.P., F.A.C.P.

Of the many topical preparations that are important in the therapy of psoriasis, probably the most widely used are corticosteroid preparations. While topical steroids are extremely valuable for some psoriatics they also have the drawback of leading to short remission of psoriasis. These agents are discussed in detail in Chapter 4.

Other agents that are valuable in the management of psoriasis are tar preparations, keratolytic agents to remove excessive scale, and emollients or moisturizers to assist in the reduction of the scaling present in many psoriatics. These other agents often have relatively weak antipsoriatic action themselves, but they are valuable as adjunctive agents when combined with other forms of therapy.

TAR PREPARATIONS

There are many different forms of tar used in the treatment of various skin diseases. The three main types are shale tars or ichthammols, wood tars, and coal tars.

Wood tars are little used in the United States but they are used in Europe. They tend to be poorly effective for treating psoriasis by themselves and are also nonphotosensitizing. They have the potential problem of contact allergic sensitization.

In this author's experience, the ichthammols or shale oil tars are relatively ineffective as topical agents for inflammatory skin diseases. They have mild occlusive and skin protectant qualities.

Coal tars have been studied extensively for their effects on different skin diseases. One major problem with coal tars is the wide variation of content, partially resulting from wide variations of the source of coal from which the coal tar is derived. Different distillation temperatures and purification procedures lead to further variation of coal tars.[8]

Coal Tar Effects on the Skin

While dermatologic therapy with coal tars has been conducted for many years, their mechanisms of action on the skin are not clearly understood. It can be shown that coal tar and coal tar products are able to suppress DNA synthesis in the epidermis within the first few hours after the application of the coal tar.[9, 14] This is somewhat similar in action to the initial suppression of epidermal DNA synthesis observed after, for example, ultraviolet-B radiation and may represent one potential mechanism of action of tars on the epidermoproliferative disease, psoriasis.

The effects of coal tars on normal skin, however, show a rather complex series of events. When coal tars are applied to normal skin there is initially suppression of epidermal DNA synthesis.[9, 14] This is followed by a proliferative response, and if the treatment is continued for as long as 40 days, following this proliferative response the tars have a subsequent cytostatic effect, with resultant epidermal thinning.[6]

It should be stressed that many of the studies with tars have been performed on normal animal or human skin[6, 8, 9, 14] or on the parakeratotic mouse tail.[16] It is quite possible that the therapeutic effects of agents such as coal tars or ultraviolet-B radiation will be different on the hyperproliferative epidermis of psoriasis. In addition to antiproliferative effects, many clinicians consider that coal tars have both anti-inflammatory and antipruritic properties.

It is also possible that coal tars correct a possible differentiation defect in psoriatic epidermis.

Pharmacological Variability of Coal Tars

Crude coal tar is the product of the distillation of bituminous coal in the absence of oxygen. Burning at very high temperatures causes the coal to undergo chemical changes that ultimately produce hundreds of new and more complex molecules in the black, viscous product called coal tar. Crude coal tar itself is a mixture of ten thousand or more components, of which fewer than half have been identified and far fewer studied for any potential therapeutic activity.[5]

Attempts that have been made to standardize production of crude coal tar for pharmaceutical use unfortunately do not seem to insure a standard product.[8] The contradiction of findings in some of the clinical studies may be due, at least in part, to variability of the coal tar composition. The epidermal DNA synthesis suppression assay utilizing the hairless mouse as an assay that appears to be predictive of antipsoriatic effectiveness of therapeutic agents.[8] The greater the ability of an agent to suppress epidermal DNA synthesis, the greater the antipsoriatic potential of such an agent.[9] In one recent study coal tars were applied to the skin of the mouse and the rates of epidermal DNA synthesis were measured. These studies showed that crude coal tar barrels obtained from the same tar supplier, collected from carbonized coal heated in excess of 970 C, showed a marked variability within the same delivered lot. The activity in the assay varied, not only between the crude coal tar fractions, but also when the crude coal tar was purified.[8]

Perhaps not surprisingly, those purified tar products produced from the originally active crude coal tar lots remained active in this assay, however, those from the originally inactive crude coal tar lots remained inactive.[8] While suppression of epidermal DNA synthesis is unlikely to be the sole therapeutic mechanism of coal tar's antipsoriatic effects, this study does provide evidence for the biologic and pharmacologic variability of coal tars even from the same supplier. (This demonstration of the variability of efficacy of different coal tars supported an impression held by some dermatologists for many years.)

Coal Tars and Phototherapy Regimens

Tar phototherapy is discussed in detail in Chapter 8; however, I will briefly discuss some controversy about whether coal tars are a necessary part of a phototherapy regimen for psoriasis treatment.

Since Goeckerman introduced the combination of ultraviolet light radiation and coal tar[4] many modifications of that combination have been suggested and studied. Recent studies[7] reported that crude coal tar was no more effective than petrolatum when combined with aggressive erythemogenic UVB radiation. They therefore questioned the need to use coal tar in this erythemogenic UVB regimen for the treatment of psoriasis.

Frost, et al.[3] had previously reported that a purified tar gel was more effective than gel base alone, when combined with suberythemogenic doses of UVB. In their study, psoriasis improved more rapidly on the tar gel–UVB-treated side compared to the gel base–UVB-treated side. This, therefore, suggested that tars contributed to the antipsoriatic effect, when used with suberythemogenic UVB radiation.

We examined these questions in further detail with both erythemogenic and suberythemogenic regimens of UVB for plaque psoriasis.[10] We used a UVB upright hexagonal cabinet containing 16 FS-72 sunlamp tubes producing their maximum emission at 313 nm. Minimal erythema dosages were determined prior to starting therapy on uninvolved areas of back skin. Our studies of patients with milder forms of psoriasis showed:

1. Erythemogenic UVB combined with 1% crude coal tar is equipotent with erythemogenic UVB and petrolatum. In other words, the psoriasis improved clinically at the same rate, on both sides of the body.

2. Suberythemogenic UVB combined with 1% crude coal tar is more effective than suberythemogenic UVB and petrolatum. In other words, the psoriasis improved more rapidly on the UVB and 1% coal tar-treated sides. Suberythemogenic UVB with purified tar body oil was more effective than suberythemogenic UVB and the oil base alone.

Potential Practical Implications for Tar and Ultraviolet Phototherapy

It is possible to obtain an ultraviolet sparing effect using an appropriately active tar preparation. Patients with mild to moderate psoriasis requiring phototherapy can be treated with a combination of tar and ultraviolet, permitting the use of smaller amounts of ultraviolet radiation. In this way fewer early side effects are seen; in particular, there is less itching, skin tenderness, and erythema produced when a suberythemogenic UVB and tar regimen is followed.

In practical terms, this usually means that patients follow the following *treatment plan.*

1. They apply a purified tar, either a tar oil or a tar gel, preferably overnight at home. If they apply this preparation and wait 10–15 minutes before dressing, the tar tends not to rub off excessively onto the bedclothes; however, it is advisable for them to use bedclothes where staining is not an important factor.

2. One compromise is to get them to apply the tar during the day and keep it on for a minimum of 2 hours before exposure to the ultraviolet radiation.

3. The patient then receives ultraviolet treatment, usually at the dermatologist's office or treatment center. The choices of ultraviolet apparatus are outlined in Chapter 7. A useful unit contains vertical UVB sunlamp tubes, which produce their maximum emission in the UVB range.

4. The patient will have his/her minimal erythema dose (MED) determined on day one on an uninvolved area of back skin that has been pre-

treated with tar preparation. The patient will then be seen the following day to have these test sites evaluated and their MED time determined. The first treatment will usually last a third of the MED time. The patient is then treated once daily as often as is possible. At each treatment the time is usually increased by one third of the MED.

There is discussion about whether the amount of ultraviolet radiation has to be constantly increased. In the author's experience, particularly with patients who have lighter skin types, it is often possible to get an adequate therapeutic response by increasing to between 3 and 5 times the MED and staying at that level. For example, if the MED is 60 seconds, ⅓ MED = 20 secs, will be the length of the first treatment, while 5 MED = 5 minutes, which will be the maximum treatment time given.

5. The frequency of therapy often depends on practicalities of transportation and work. In the author's experience, unless the patient is able to be treated at least three times weekly, the therapeutic response is poor in the early treatment phase. There are some patients after maximum improvement or clearance with this modified outpatient regimen with tar and ultraviolet who are able to be maintained with once weekly or less frequent maintenance therapy.

It should be stressed that this form of treatment usually is practical for less severely affected psoriasis patients; patients with more extensive or more resistant psoriasis usually need more intensive forms of therapy, involving the use of modified Goeckerman treatments and anthralin in a daycare or hospital setting. We are not certain about the long-term toxicity of this type of treatment compared to more aggressive ultraviolet treatment not using coal tars. It is, however, expected that it would be at least as safe as the standard Goeckerman program.

Coal Tars Used Without Phototherapy

Evidence for the potential direct effect of coal tars on the epidermis is from the studies showing the cytostatic effect of tars on the epidermis after long-term usage.[6] In addition, the finding that coal tar preparations suppressed epidermal DNA synthesis in the hairless mouse[8, 14] suggests a potential effect on psoriasis. We reexamined this question using a purified coal tar oil in some patients with chronic plaque psoriasis. When the tar-containing oil was applied daily to lesions on one side of the body and the oil without tar to the other side, a significantly greater response was achieved in the tar-treated sides (Plate 1).[10]

These studies, therefore, confirm that under these experimental conditions, a tar oil was more effective than the oil base alone. The tar preparation used in these studies was T-Derm Tar Oil.®

Practical Aspects of Coal Tar Usage in Psoriasis

There are several situations where coal tar preparations are extremely valuable as adjunctive agents in the treatment of psoriasis. The combination of coal tars with ultraviolet phototherapy is discussed in Chapter 8. In this author's experience, it is often valuable to combine coal tar preparations with topical corticosteroids and with anthralin therapy on an outpatient, day-care or inpatient basis.

For example, a possible treatment program for localized psoriasis consists of the patient applying a topical corticosteroid cream or ointment once or twice daily. At night he or she applies a purified tar preparation, allowing the tar to dry on the skin for at least 10–15 minutes prior to bed, minimizing staining of the bedclothes. An alternative program is for the patient to apply anthralin as a short-contact program at home, either first thing in the morning or in the early evening, followed 15–30 minutes later by a shower. This program is discussed in more detail in Chapter 6. Before bed the patient may apply one of the purified tar preparations, some of which are listed in Table 5–1.

Side Effects of Coal Tars Seen During Therapy

One main problem with tars is their relative messiness. Even the purified tar preparations stain clothing if the patient does not allow time for as much as possible of the tar preparation to absorb into the skin.

In addition to this problem, coal tars produce folliculitis in some patients. This may be more of a problem with concentrations above equivalent 2% crude coal tar and also with some of the more occlusive ointment bases (e.g., petrolatum).

In the author's experience, if folliculitis occurs a less occlusive base can be used, such as Eucerin or Aquaphor. A lower concentration of crude coal tar (for example, 1%) can be used in this situation, or the crude coal tar substituted with 5% or 10% liquor carbonis detergens (LCD). There is less risk of folliculitis with some of the purified tar preparations listed in Table 5–1.

Patient instructions should point out the potential problems of coal tar use (Table 5–2).

TABLE 5–1.—SOME COMMERCIAL
PURIFIED TAR PREPARATIONS AVAILABLE
IN THE UNITED STATES FOR THE THERAPY
OF BODY AND SCALP PSORIASIS

Baker's P and S Plus Gel
Estar Tar Gel
Fototar Tar Cream
Psorigel
T-Derm Tar Oil
T-Derm Tar and Salicylic Acid Scalp Lotion
Also available as an alternative to crude coal tar:
  Liquor carbonis detergens, usually between
    5% to 20% concentrations in cream,
    ointment or oil.
Also available as an additive for bathwater:
  Balnetar
  Doak oil

Possible Delayed Side Effects of Coal Tars

There recently has been a study showing that coal tar treated psoriatic patients percutaneously absorb and excrete from their urine mutagenic substances.[15] The concentrations of these urinary mutagens in nonsmoking psoriatics were, however, much lower than those excreted from patients who were cigarette smokers. The significance of these absorbed coal tar derived mutagens is unclear at present, because some recent retrospective studies have failed to show an increased incidence of skin cancer or systemic cancers in tar-treated patients.[11] A further study by Stern, et al.[12] showed that in some of their patients treatment with tar and ultraviolet light resulted in a small increased risk of developing skin cancer. The patients at greater risk appeared to be those with lighter skin types.

Further, long-term studies are desirable to determine safety of long-term usage of tar body preparations.

TABLE 5–2.—COAL TAR PRODUCTS FOR PSORIASIS: PATIENT INSTRUCTIONS

Many of these products can be messy and *stain* your clothing and furnishings.
Apply *small amounts* and rub them well into the skin. Use old or stained garments as clothing after applying the coal tars.
Many purified tar gels, lotions, creams, or oils will cease staining your clothes after they have been on the skin for several minutes.
Avoid any sun exposure of coal tar-treated skin unless advised by your physician. He may advise sun or ultraviolet treatments after you apply the coal tar, but these have to be done with his advice to avoid skin burning.
If *skin infections, infections* around hairs, increased redness of the skin, or stinging or smarting of the skin occurs, *stop* using the coal tar until you have checked with your physician.

Coal Tar Therapy: Conclusions

1. There is significant evidence for the effectiveness of tars as antipso-riatic therapy.

2. When used alone, coal tars are weakly antipsoriatic, and do not have the efficacy of anthralin or potent topical steroids.

3. However, when combined with certain phototherapy regimens they appear to be useful agents. It appears that some coal tars in combination with suberythemogenic UVB are a useful and effective treatment for pso-riasis.

4. It remains to be seen whether such a combination is potentially less hazardous to the skin than greater amounts of UVB erythemogenic radia-tion, without the tar.

KERATOLYTICS

Keratolytics are agents that help to remove the diseased scale or hyper-keratosis in psoriasis and other diseases. Their precise mechanism of action is not known,[1] but they are valuable as part of a psoriasis treatment pro-gram, particularly in those patients who have scaling psoriasis.

Salicylic Acid

Topical salicylic acid is the most frequently used keratolytic agent. It may be used alone or, more commonly, in conjunction with other forms of therapy.

The concentration range usually used for salicylic acid is between 2% and 10%. Caution is to be exercised when this agent is applied extensively to the body, particularly in children, since use may result in salicylism.[2] Symptoms include tinnitus, nausea, and hyperventilation.

Very rarely, if there is marked hyperkeratosis, for example, on the knees, elbows, palms or soles, short-term use of up to 20% salicylic acid in a cream or ointment base can be used for a few days. If these concentra-tions are used for too long a period of time, maceration of the skin can occur.

Salicylic acid, as noted, is often combined with other forms of therapy, most frequently with coal tar preparations, including crude coal tar and LCD. These combinations are particularly useful in the early stages of topical therapy for the patient with more scaling psoriasis. In the author's practice, these agents are used for enough time to clear the scale and then a nonsalicylic acid-containing tar preparation is substituted; for example, when Goeckerman or modified Goeckerman therapy is being used. A commercially available preparation of salicylic acid gel (Keralyt, in the United States) is convenient to use and may be mixed with one of the tar gels for the home treatment of some selected psoriasis patients. This combination is also useful for scalp psoriasis.

Other Stratum Corneum Modifying Agents

Other topical agents that have been described as having a possible keratolytic effect are the alpha-hydroxy acids. These have been used particularly in patients with ichthyosis.[13] They include lactic acid, tartaric acid, pyruvic acid, and glycolic acid. There is a high-concentration lactic acid lotion that may be available in the United States in 1985. This may be useful in the treatment of some hyperkeratotic disorders, including ichthyosis and psoriasis.

Another group of topical agents that the author finds particularly useful for hyperkeratotic psoriasis are the urea-containing preparations. Ten percent urea, which may also be formulated with topical corticosteroids or anthralin, is often useful to prescribe for some psoriatics. One practical problem with the use of some urea preparations is the stinging sensation that can occur when applied to skin. In the author's experience, if the urea preparation is applied shortly after bathing the degree of stinging is reduced and can be tolerated by the patient. Among the urea-containing preparations available commercially is Carmol®. Urea-hydrocortisone preparations include Carmol-hydrocortisone® and Alphaderm® cream.

EMOLLIENTS

Emollients are topical agents that smooth and soften the stratum corneum. They are particularly useful in situations where excessive drying or accumulation of stratum corneum occurs. These situations include psoriasis and ichthyosis as well as common problems such as dry skin and certain categories of eczema.

It is thought that most emollients have their effect, not by rehydration of the stratum corneum, but by a trapping mechanism that slows down the rate of transepidermal water loss. In general, the more occlusive the emollient, the more effective it will be. For example, petrolatum U.S.P. is a very effective emollient. In the author's practice patients are encouraged to find an emollient that they are willing and able to use on a regular basis. They apply these agents as frequently as is practical during the day, usually no more than twice daily. An important time for application of emollient is after bathing or showering. The patient will pat-dry the skin and gently apply the emollient, then wait and wear a loose gown to allow the emollient to have some effect and not be immediately removed by rubbing on clothing.

The most practical way of getting patients to use emollients is to provide them with the names of several alternative agents that can be obtained from the pharmacy, and perhaps to provide samples. Some available emollients are listed in Table 5–3. When patients have found the emollient that they are able to use, they may use it on a routine basis.

Contents of Emollients

The ingredients of emollients vary considerably. Mineral oils are probably the most commonly used emollient oils. Other less commonly used oils

TABLE 5–3.—SOME SELECTED
EMOLLIENTS

Acid Mantle Creme & Lotion
Alpha Keri Shower and Bath Oil
Aquaphor Cream
Carmol 10 Lotion
Carmol 20 Cream
Complex 15 Moisturizing Cream & Lotion
Eucerin Creme
Eucerin Lotion
Lubriderm Cream
Lubriderm Lotion
Lubriderm Lubath Bath Shower Oil
Neutrogena Norwegian Formula Hand Cream
Neutrogena Facial Moisturizer
Neutrogena Body Oil
Neutrogena Lotion for Hand & Body
Petrolatum White U.S.P.
pHisoDerm
Purpose Dry Skin Cream
Shepard's Cream Lotion
Shepard's Skin Cream
Shepard's Soap
Vaseline Dermatology Formula Cream
Vaseline Dermatology Formula Lotion
Vaseline Pure Petroleum Jelly Skin Protectant

include a variety of vegetable oils, such as sunflower seed oil. Oils of animal origin, and in particular whale oil, have tended for a variety of reasons to be used less frequently, particularly in the United States. Lanolin is still used occasionally, but there are concerns of lanolin sensitivity. Other agents include urea, glycerin, and petrolatum.

Emollients as a Necessary Component of Phototherapy Treatment

It has been shown that the use of an emollient such as petrolatum can enhance the effects of UVB phototherapy for psoriasis.[7] In this study, patients treated with UVB therapy had a better response in skin areas where petrolatum was supplied than in areas of skin that were treated with phototherapy alone. The possible reasons for this include enhanced penetration and therapeutic effect of the ultraviolet on the epidermis. One possible mechanism of this is alteration of the optical and UV-transmitting properties of the stratum corneum by the application of the emollient.

This is of practical importance, and in the author's treatment center all patients who have any significant scaling over their psoriatic areas have an emollient, usually petrolatum, applied immediately prior to phototherapy, whether UVB or PUVA. This enhances the effectiveness of the phototherapy.

The choice of emollient has to be particularly critical in some situations. In hairy patients excessively occlusive emollients may produce folliculitis. On the back and on the face certain emollients aggravate or cause acneiform eruptions. There are many commercially available emollients that are claimed to be noncomedogenic, and in the author's experience it is wise always to use these agents on the face and chest of patients who have a history of acne in those areas.

Use of Emollients: Conclusions

1. Emollients are a most important component of therapy for psoriasis.

2. They are particularly valuable in patients with dry skin and skin dryness aggravated by frequent bathing and phototherapy.

3. They appear to enhance the efficacy of phototherapy, possibly by altering the optical and UV-transmitting characteristics of the stratum corneum.

4. There is great personal patient preference for different emollients; it

is advised that several names or samples be given and patients be allowed to find the emollient that they are willing and able to use on a regular basis.

REFERENCES

1. Davies M., Marks R.: Studies on the effects of salicylic acid on normal skin. *Br. J. Dermatol.* 95:187–192, 1976.
2. Davies M.G., Briffa D.V., Greaves M.W.: Systemic toxicity from topically applied salicylic acid. *Br. Med. J.* 1:661, 1979.
3. Frost P., Horwitz S.N., Caputo R.V., et al.: Tar gel-phototherapy for psoriasis. *Arch. Dermatol.* 115:840–846, 1979.
4. Goeckerman W.H.: Treatment of Psoriasis. *Northwest Med.* 24:229–231, 1925.
5. Grupper C.: The chemistry, pharmacology and use of tar in the treatment of psoriasis, in Farber E.M., Cox A.J. (eds.): *Psoriasis, Proceedings of International Symposium.* Stanford Press, 1971, p. 347, Palo Alto, Calif.
6. Lavker R.M., Grove G.L., Kligman A.M.: The atrophogenic effect of crude coal tar on human epidermis. *Br. J. Dermatol.* 105:77–82, 1981.
7. Levine M.J., White H.A.D., Parrish J.A.: Components of the Goeckerman regimen. *J. Invest. Dermatol.* 73:170–173, 1979.
8. Lowe N.J., Breeding J., Wortzman M.S.: The pharmacological variability of crude coal tar. *Br. J. Dermatol.* 107:475–480, 1982.
9. Lowe N.J., Stoughton R.B., McCullough J.L., et al.: Topical drugs on normal and proliferating epidermal cell models; comparison with responses in psoriatics. *Arch. Dermatol.* 117:394–398, 1981.
10. Lowe N.J., Wortzman M.S., Breeding J., et al.: Coal tar phototherapy for psoriasis re-evaluated. *J. Am. Acad. Dermatol.* 8:781–789, 1983.
11. Pettelkow M.R., Perry H.O., Mueller S.A., et al.: Skin cancer in patients undergoing coal tar therapy for psoriasis. *J. Int. Derm.* 77:181–185, 1981.
12. Stern R.S., Zietler S., Parrish J.A.: Skin carcinoma in outpatients treated with topical tar and artificial ultraviolet radiation. *Lancet* 1:732–734, 1980.
13. Van Scott E.J., Yu R.J.: Control of keratinization with alpha-hydroxy acids and related compounds: I. Topical treatment of ichthyotic disorders. *Arch. Dermatol.* 110:586–590, 1974.
14. Walter J.F., Stoughton R.B., DeQuoy P.R.: Suppression of epidermal DNA synthesis by ultraviolet light, coal tar and anthralin. *Br. J. Dermatol.* 99:89–96, 1978.
15. Wheeler L., Lowe N.J.: Mutagenicity of urines from patients undergoing coal tar therapy for psoriasis. *J. Invest. Dermatol.* 77:181–185, 1981.
16. Wrench R., Britten Z.: Evaluation of coal tar fractions in psoriasiform diseases using the mouse tail test. *Br. J. Dermatol.* 92:569–574, 1975.

6 / Anthralin Use in the Treatment of Psoriasis

Richard E. Ashton, M.B., M.R.C.P.
Nicholas J. Lowe, M.D., F.R.C.P., F.A.C.P.

ANTHRALIN (Fig 6–1) is a synthetic derivative of anthracene. It was first produced in Germany in 1916 and was derived from a natural product, chrysarobin. This was the active constituent of Goa powder, a herbal remedy derived from the bark of the South American araroba tree. Goa powder originally had been used to treat ringworm, but Balmanno Squire, a British dermatologist, discovered its effectiveness in psoriasis.[2] Anthralin has been extensively used in Europe and in Britain,[8] but its use in the United States has taken second place to topical steroids and to tar and ultraviolet light in the treatment of psoriasis.[7]

FORMULATIONS

Anthralin is a yellow powder, soluble in organic solvents. It is easily oxidized in air to the anthraquinone, anthralin dimer, and anthralin conjugates,[3] which are colored varying shades of brown. Anthralin formulations can therefore easily become degraded. Anthralin must be dissolved in petrolatum initially, but the solubility is low, around 2%, the rest existing as a suspension. A more uniform mixture is obtained by first dissolving the anthralin in chloroform and adding this to the petrolatum. The chloroform is allowed to evaporate off, leaving the suspension in petrolatum.

Anthralin ointment may be prepared by any pharmacy, but it is also available commercially in 0.1%, 0.25%, 0.5%, and 1.0% concentrations. Anthralin cream consists of an oil-in-water emulsion, with anthralin dissolved in the oily phase and salicylic acid in the water phase to prevent

40

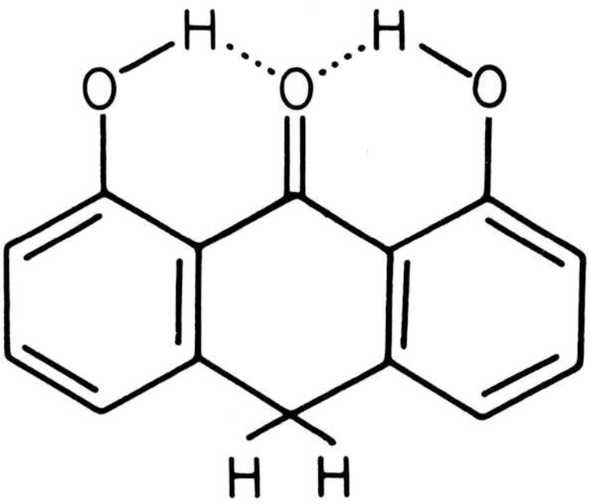

Fig 6–1.—Chemical structure of anthralin.

oxidation of the anthralin. This is marketed in 0.1%, 0.25%, 0.5%, and 1.0% strengths. Anthralin paste contains varying strengths of anthralin in Lassar's paste, which contains zinc oxide, starch, salicylic acid, and petrolatum. Anthralin sticks are available. The anthralin is suspended in beeswax. Since delivery of anthralin from the stick is not as high as from petrolatum higher strengths need to be used, usually either 1% or 2%.

SIDE EFFECTS OF ANTHRALIN

Skin Irritation

Before using anthralin, both patient and physician should be aware of the only two side effects, skin irritation and staining of clothing and normal skin. On the skin, anthralin is oxidized and these oxidation products can combine with proteins in the stratum corneum to produce the typical brown staining[1] (Fig 6–2). The anthralin-generated superoxide radical, which is probably responsible for its therapeutic effect, is also capable of initiating an inflammatory response.[4] Patients vary in their ability to tolerate anthralin, and this toleration is usually strength-dependent. Some patients cannot tolerate strengths as low as 0.1%, while others may tolerate more than 4%.

Skin Staining

Patients should be encouraged to identify anthralin staining as a sign of progress in treatment. In addition, it can alert the physician as to whether

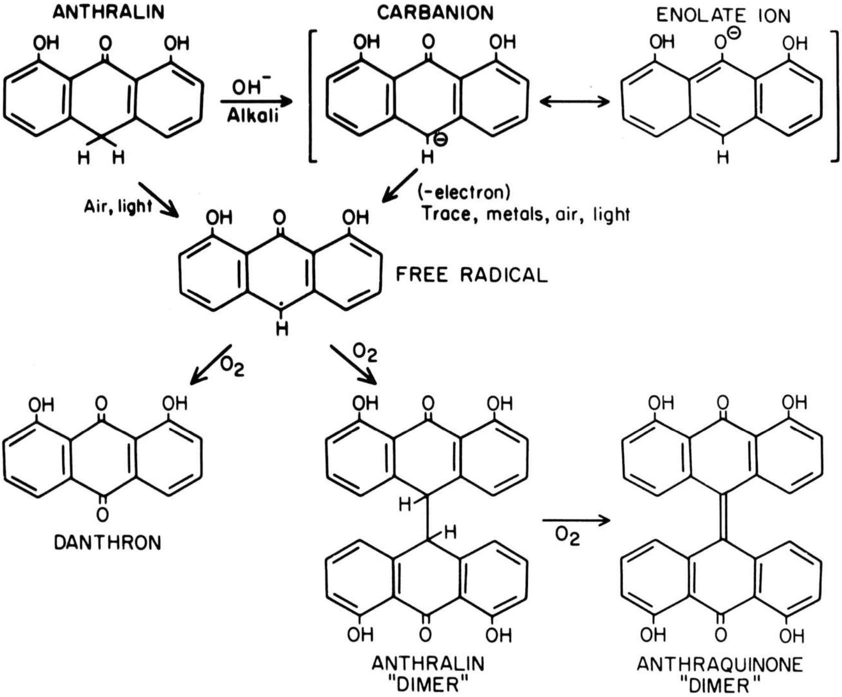

Fig 6–2.—Oxidation of anthralin to the free radical and other colored derivatives responsible for anthralin staining. (Modified from Krebbs A., et al.[3])

the patient has been using the medication effectively. Only the surrounding skin will stain initially, while the psoriatic plaques do not stain due to the high turnover of the stratum corneum. Eventually, presumably when the epidermal cell turnover is reduced as the psoriasis is clearing, the plaque itself takes up the stain. The stain usually clears two to three weeks after stopping treatment (Fig 6–3).

Treatment of the stained skin with a keratolytic agent such as salicylic acid will help to hasten the removal of stained stratum corneum.

ANTHRALIN PREPARATIONS

Anthralin preparations are available in a variety of forms and concentrations, as summarized in Table 6–1.

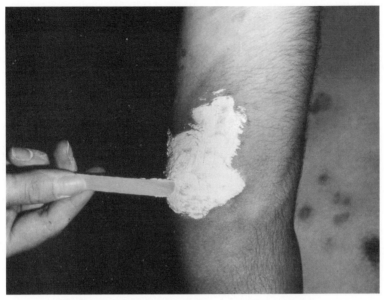

Fig 6–3.—Applying anthralin paste with a spatula.

Anthralin Ointment

This may be rubbed onto psoriatic areas. The disadvantage with the ointment preparation is that it tends to spread off the plaque onto normal skin, making irritation of the normal skin more likely. In addition, ointments remain on the surface and can stain clothing. It seems that the minimum effective concentration for anthralin to clear extensive plaque psoriasis in an ointment base is 0.1%.[5] Anthralin ointment is effective when used following the short-contact therapy method.[13] Some available anthralin ointment preparations are listed in Table 6–2.

Anthralin Paste

To prevent the anthralin from spreading off the psoriatic plaques, Lassar's paste, which tends to remain on the plaques, can be applied. The disadvantages of this therapy are that it requires nurses skilled in its application, and its removal is difficult. In addition, patients have to wear special suits over the skin to protect clothing. In spite of these disadvantages, anthralin paste therapy (Ingram's regimen) provides for rapid clearance of

TABLE 6–1.—SOME AVAILABLE ANTHRALIN PREPARATIONS
WITH USUAL CONCENTRATIONS

FORM OF PREPARATION	PRODUCT NAME	MANUFACTURER	CONCENTRATIONS (%)
Paste	Formulated by pharmacist in Lassar's paste (see text)		0.1–5.0
Ointment	See Table 6–2		
Cream	Dithrocream†	Dermal (U.K.)	0.1, 0.25, 0.5
	Drithocream*	Dermal (U.S.A.)	0.1, 0.25, 0.5, 1.0
	Lasan*	Stiefel (U.S.A.)	0.1, 0.2, 0.4, 1.0
	Anthranol‡	Stiefel (Canada)	0.1, 0.2, 0.4
	Psoradrate†	Eaton	0.1, 0.2
Stick	Anthraderm†	Brocades	0.5, 1.0
	(Unnamed)*	Westwood	1.0
Future options: Solutions Gels Tapes Possibility of effective Anthralin analogues			

*Available in United States.
†Available in United Kingdom.
‡Available in Canada.

TABLE 6–2.—ANTHRALIN OINTMENT
PREPARATIONS AVAILABLE COMMERCIALLY

U.S.:
Anthraderm (Dermik) 0.1%, 0.25%, 0.5%, 1.0%
Lassan (Stiefel) 0.1%, 0.25%, 0.5%, 1.0%
Britain:
Stie Lassan (Stiefel) Dithranol 0.4%, salicylic acid 0.4%
Anthranol 0.4%, 1.0%, 2.0%
Canada:
Lassan (Stiefel) 0.1%, 0.25%, 0.5%, 1.0%

the psoriasis (average three weeks). Since the 1950s it has been the treatment of choice, combined often with tar baths and ultraviolet, for inpatient psoriasis therapy in Britain.[8] Its use is probably best restricted to inpatient or day-care centers. The full details of Ingram's regimen are given later in this chapter.

Anthralin Cream

One anthralin cream preparation was formulated as a vanishing cream. Cream has the advantage over the ointment that it can be rubbed in. Provided the excess is wiped off the skin with a tissue, anthralin staining and

TABLE 6–3.—ANTHRALIN CREAM PREPARATIONS
AVAILABLE COMMERCIALLY

U.S.:
Drithocream (American Dermal) 0.1%, 0.25%, 0.5%, 1.0%
Britain:
Dithrocream (Dermal) 0.1%, 0.25%, 0.5%
Psoradrate (Easton) 0.1%, 0.2% in 17% urea cream
Anthranol (Stiefel) 0.1%, 0.2%, 0.4%

---

irritation may be minimized.[9, 10] This also can be used in the short-contact therapy method of anthralin therapy.[18] (T. Kingston and N.J. Lowe, Unpublished studies, 1984). A list of available anthralin cream preparations is given in Table 6–3.

Anthralin Sticks

These are useful for isolated plaques of psoriasis, such as on elbows and knees, where patients want to apply small amounts of anthralin accurately.[11] The sticks have the advantage that they are acceptable to patients, minimizing hand contact with the anthralin. The sticks probably do not produce such rapid clearance as properly applied ointments or creams, but they are effective as short-contact treatments.[20] Table 6–4 lists commercially available anthralin stick preparations.

ANTHRALIN TREATMENT PROGRAMS

Ingram's Regimen

Ingram in Leeds, England, developed an effective method of using anthralin by adding anthralin paste to the Goeckerman regimen.[8]

TABLE 6–4.—ANTHRALIN STICK
PREPARATIONS AVAILABLE COMMERCIALLY

U.S.:
(Not available as of October 1984) Westwood
    Pharmaceuticals is expected to have 1% anthralin
    stick available in 1985 or 1986.
Britain:
Antraderm (Brocades) 0.5%, 1.0%

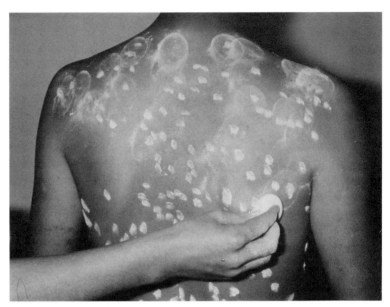

Fig 6–4.—Dabbing powder over the applied paste.

The treatment consists of the following:[8]

1. The patient has a tar bath for about 15–30 minutes with a coal tar solution (such as Balnetar, Zetar, or Polytar) added to the bathwater.

2. Following this, the skin is exposed to suberythemogenic doses of broad-range ultraviolet light using a mercury vapor lamp. Nowadays, several predominantly UVB sources may be used, perhaps the most convenient being a cabinet of Westinghouse sunlamp (FS) tubes. The dose can be increased at each treatment, provided no burning occurs. Start with one third of a minimal erythema dose and increase by this amount with each therapy. The peak ultraviolet emission with these FS tubes is at 313 mm, but they also emit some UVA and UVC radiation.

3. Anthralin paste is applied with a spatula to all psoriatic plaques at an initial dose of 0.1%. The anthralin in Lassar's paste should be soft enough to be spread easily with a spatula or tongue depressor. It is important to apply the paste only to the psoriatic plaques, sparing normal skin (Fig 6–4). The next highest concentration (initially 0.25%) is applied to a test area.

4. The paste is powdered with talc. It is convenient to make a powder ball, using gauze, so the talc may be conveniently dabbed onto the treated area (Fig 6–5). The talc removes any moisture from the paste and prevents staining of clothing.

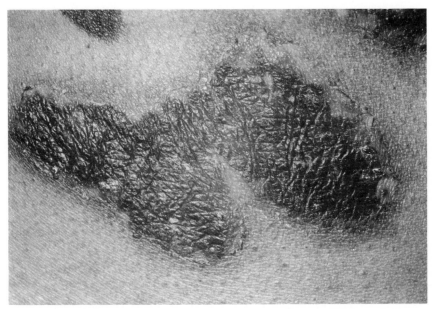

Fig 6–5.—Nonscaly plaque after removal of the paste.

5. The whole body may be covered in a tubular netting suit. Holes have to be cut for arms and the netting around the arms and legs attached to that around the trunk using ties.

6. The anthralin paste may be left on for periods varying from six to 24 hours. Except in a psoriasis day-care setting, it is convenient to leave the paste in place for a day. Prior to bathing, the paste must be removed with liquid paraffin. Cotton balls are soaked in the liquid paraffin and rubbed onto the paste to remove it. In addition to the paste the excessive scaling is removed, leaving a clean psoriatic plaque (Fig 6–6).

7. The procedure is repeated with a tar bath, then exposure to UVL, and finally application of the paste at a higher concentration. Usually concentrations can be increased on alternate days (Table 6–5). The rate of increase of both UVL and anthralin paste must remain flexible and may be determined by whether the patient experiences any side effects of irritation. Should this occur, the dose should not be increased and may need to be reduced. If severe burning from UVL occurs, light treatment must be suspended. Anthralin burning will also require temporary discontinuation of the paste and treatment with petrolatum. Once the irritation has subsided, anthralin paste may be restarted but at a lower dose.

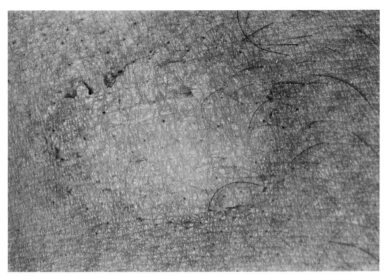

Fig 6–6.—Hypopigmented area after completion of treatment and removal of anthralin staining.

Short-Contact Therapy

This recent modification of anthralin therapy has made outpatient anthralin a much easier therapy than before. It is possible that anthralin is absorbed more rapidly into psoriatic skin than normal skin. Thus, if a high concentration is applied for a short period of time and then removed, rel-

TABLE 6–5.—RECOMMENDED STRENGTH INCREASE
OF ANTHRALIN PASTE IN THE INGRAM REGIMEN*

DAY	%
1	0.1
3	0.25
5	0.5
7	0.75
9	1.0
11	2.0
13	3.0
15	4.0

*If skin irritation occurs, reduce to next lower concentration for 2–3 days and then again try to increase concentration after irritation has resolved. Some patients improve dramatically with low concentrations, others need 4% or higher to achieve good responses.

TABLE 6–6.—PATIENT INFORMATION SHEET FOR HOME USE OF ANTHRALIN
SHORT-CONTACT THERAPY

1. Apply anthralin cream/ointment/stick only to psoriasis. Do not apply to normal skin. You may prefer to use plastic disposable gloves to apply the anthralin to avoid staining the hands and nails.
2. Anthralin should be rubbed in well and any excess wiped off. You should wash the skin with soap and shower after 15 or 30 minutes.
3. Anthralin will stain a brown to purple color. Use old clothing and sheets when anthralin is on the skin. If staining occurs rinse with water (do not soap).
4. Expect to see a brown stain on normal surrounding skin after using anthralin. This is a good sign and indicates that the anthralin is working. When the stain occurs in the center the psoriasis is clearing.
5. Should irritation or burning occur on the skin, stop using the anthralin until it settles. Then restart application cautiously at a lower strength.
6. If no irritation or burning occurs on the skin, the contact time may increase to 1 hour and then the anthralin strength may be increased weekly. Start at 0.1% and increase to 0.25%, 0.5% and 1%.
7. The psoriasis is clear when it cannot be felt, even though the brown stain is present. Stop treatment and the stain will clear in 1–2 weeks.
8. Wash hands after applying anthralin. Do not rub eyes with anthralin-contaminated fingers. Do not apply anthralin near eyes.
9. Should eye irritation occur, irrigate eyes with water and consult your doctor.

atively more of the anthralin will penetrate the psoriatic skin as compared to normal surrounding skin. The effect of this treatment is to increase effectiveness of anthralin and reduce the side effects of skin irritation and staining.[6, 12, 13] By leaving the anthralin on for short periods, staining of clothing can be avoided. The treatment can be carried out at home (Table 6–6) and old garments worn during the treatment. The anthralin is then washed off the skin with soap in a shower.

Either anthralin cream or ointment may be used in short-contact therapy. These initially should be left on for 15 minutes, but if tolerated can be left on for up to an hour. If anthralin cream is used, it is best to start with the 0.25% or 0.5% strength, increasing to the 1.0% strength. The anthralin cream may be removed by gently wiping with a tissue, or washed off with liquid soap in a bath or shower.

Anthralin ointments have one advantage over the cream in that strengths greater than 1% can be prepared by some pharmacists. Initially it is best to start with the 0.25% or 0.5% strengths, but this may be increased to 4%. One study found that 4% anthralin left on for 15 minutes produces the most rapid results. The anthralin ointment should be removed in a shower or bath with liquid soap.

Anthralin Treatment of the Scalp

Scalp psoriasis is often a problem to control. Frequent application of steroid lotions or washing with tar-based shampoos often does not clear thick scales that accumulate on the scalp of some psoriatics. Anthralin pomade is often helpful. It must be made up by a pharmacy and consists of the following:

Anthralin (1%), salicylic acid (0.4%), mineral oil (74.6%), cetyl alcohol (21.9%), and sodium lauryl sulphate (2.1%).

The pomade should be massaged onto the scalp at night and left in place overnight. The following morning it is removed by washing the hair with a regular shampoo. The treatment should be applied as often as necessary to clear thick scales or maintain clearance. This initially can be daily, but less frequent application, on a weekly or twice-weekly basis, is often sufficient.

An alternative is to use one of the anthralin creams for short contact periods followed by thorough shampooing.

Anthralin may also be formulated in propylene glycol as a lotion. It is most important to warn patients to avoid eye contamination when treating the scalp.

Combination With Other Treatments

In addition to using anthralin preparations as described, they may also be used in combination with other forms of therapy to attempt to achieve more rapid clearing. Examples include topical steroids, PUVA,[14, 15] and systemic retinoids.[16, 17]

Summary of Anthralin Therapy

Patient instruction is vital. Short-contact therapy is a practical home or outpatient therapy. Prolonged remissions are possible.

REFERENCES

1. Ashton R.E., Andre P., Lowe N.J., et al.: Anthralin: historical and current perspectives. *J. Am. Acad. Dermatol.* 9:173–192, 1983.
2. Squire B.: Treatment of psoriasis by an ointment of chrysophanic acid. *Br. Med. J.* 2:819–820, 1876.

3. Krebbs A., Shaltegger H., Shaltegger A.: Structure specificity of the antipsoriatic anthrones. *Br. J. Dermatol.* 105(Suppl 20):6–11, 1981.
4. Whitefield M.: Pharmaceutical formulations of anthralin. *Br. J. Dermatol.* 105(Suppl. 20):28–32, 1981.
5. Lowe N.J., Breeding J.: Anthralin, different concentration effects on epidermal cell DNA synthesis rates in mice and clinical responses in human psoriasis. *Arch. Dermatol.* 117:698–700, 1981.
6. Schaefer H., Farber E.M., Goldberg L., et al.: Limited application period for dithranol in psoriasis: Preliminary report on penetration and clinical efficacy. *Br. J. Dermatol.* 102:571–573, 1980.
7. Goeckerman W.H.: The treatment of psoriasis. *Northwest. Med.* 24:229–331, 1925.
8. Ingram J.T.: The approach to psoriasis. *Br. Med. J.* 2:591–594, 1953.
9. Seville R.H., Walker G.B., Whitefield M.: Dithranol cream. *Br. J. Dermatol.* 100:457–458, 1979.
10. Wilson P.D., Ive F.A.: Dithocream in psoriasis. *Br. J. Dermatol.* 102:105–106, 1980.
11. Brandt H., Mustakallio K.K.: Improved application of dithranol for ambulatory treatment of psoriasis, in Farber E.M., Cox A.J. (eds): *Proceedings of the Third International Symposium on Psoriasis*. New York, Grune & Stratton Inc., 1981, pp. 385–386.
12. Runne U., Kunze J.: Short-duration ("minutes") therapy with dithranol for psoriasis: A new out-patient regimen. *Br. J. Dermatol.* 106:135–139, 1982.
13. Lowe N.J., Ashton R.E., Koudsi H., et al.: Anthralin for psoriasis: Short contact anthralin therapy compared with topical steroid and conventional anthralin. *J. Am. Acad. Dermatol.* 10:69–72, 1984.
14. Morison W.L., Parrish J.A., Fitzpatrick T.B.: Controlled study of PUVA and adjunctive topical therapy in the management of psoriasis. *Br. J. Dermatol.* 98:125–132, 1978.
15. Cripps D.J., Lowe N.J.: Photochemotherapy for psoriasis remission times. Psoralens and UV-A and combined photochemotherapy with anthralin. *Clin. Exp. Dermatol.* 4:477–483, 1979.
16. Orfanos C.E., Runne U.: Systemic use of a new retinoid with and without local dithranol treatment in generalised psoriasis. *Br. J. Dermatol.* 95:101–103, 1976.
17. Moy R., Ashton R.E., Lowe N.J.: 13-cis-retinoic acid therapy for psoriasis. Good response in generalized pustular psoriasis, less effective than etretinate for plaque psoriasis. Manuscript submitted for publication, 1984.
18. Kingston T., Lowe N.J.: Unpublished studies, 1984.
19. Lowe N.J., Kingston T.: Unpublished studies, 1984.

7 / Phototherapy Equipment: Selection of Apparatus

Thomas F. Anderson, M.D.

It is becoming increasingly evident that ultraviolet light phototherapy is the treatment of choice for a subpopulation of patients with moderate-to-severe psoriasis. As our sophistication and understanding of the nuances of phototherapy protocols increase, it is clear that natural sunlight and suntanning parlors are *not* the appropriate sources of this treatment. Sunlight, despite its financial advantage, is limited by the vagaries of weather, lack of privacy, and temptation to utilize in a relatively ineffective way with only once- or twice-weekly exposures. Suntan parlors are operated by medically unsophisticated personnel, utilizing equipment not approved for medical use by the FDA, often with ultraviolet light sources producing longer wavelength radiation not designed for psoriasis phototherapy, at considerable medical/legal risk.[6, 13, 26]

Dermatologists are now being asked, more than ever before, to evaluate and recommend apparatus to hospitals, physiotherapists, and patients (for home use). Phototherapy protocols and equipment have changed dramatically in the last 30 years.[3, 5, 14] Increasing numbers of dermatologists are evaluating and purchasing phototherapy equipment for their offices. With the virtual explosion of phototherapy equipment manufacturers and treatment protocols, what is the practicing clinician to do?

The purpose of this chapter is to acquaint the practitioner with the range of phototherapy apparatus available and to discuss what medical practice and equipment factors are important in the evaluation and comparison of these radiation sources. In addition, the uses and sources of other adjunctive phototherapy equipment will be discussed, including radiometers, eye protection equipment, and apparatus needed to do ultraviolet light testing.

DEFINITIONS[5, 12, 14, 20]

Before proceeding, a short review of some terms important to the understanding of phototherapy, ultraviolet light sources and dosimetry is necessary.

Radiant light sources used in photomedicine deliver electromagnetic radiation (photons), generally between 200 and 4,000 nm. Those important in the phototherapy of psoriasis (Table 7–1) produce radiation between 250 and 400 nm. Germicidal ultraviolet light type C (UVC: 200–280 nm) appears to have little or no application in the treatment of psoriasis. Ultraviolet light type B (UVB: 280–320 nm) and type A (UVA: 320–400 nm) are therapeutically important in a wide variety of modified Goeckerman[4, 14, 18] and psoralen photochemotherapy protocols,[2, 14] respectively.

Dosimetry is the measurement of radiant energy delivered in a treatment protocol per unit surface area. This is usually specified as energy per square centimeter of body surface for a given wave band of radiation. *Radiometers* are devices that measure radiant energy per unit area per unit time (Energy = Power × Time). This measured *intensity, irradiance,* or *fluence* is the power of the radiant light source per unit area. For example, one Watt per square meter (W/sq m) equals 100 microwatts per square centimeter (μW/sq cm). A typical *dose* of phototherapeutic radiation is equal to the product of the intensity of the source multiplied by the time of exposure recorded as energy per unit area; for example: milliwatt seconds per square centimeter (mW sec/sq cm) or millijoules per square centimeter (mJ/sq cm). One important dose in phototherapy protocols for psoriasis is the *minimum erythema dose* (MED), defined as that dose of radiation (usually determined by titration) which produces a minimally perceptible (delayed) erythema for defined conditions (e.g., light source, skin type, distance, and time course). Commonly, for skin types I–III, a typical MED would be 20–30 mJ/sq cm of UVB (e.g., 12–25 minutes of noontime summer sun in the northeast United States). A comparable term is the *minimum phototoxic dose* (MPD), used for psoralen photochemotherapy, defined for PUVA as the dose of UVA delivered two hours after the ingestion of psoralen necessary to produce minimally perceptible (delayed) erythema.

Two other important terms used to describe typical radiation sources used in the treatment of psoriasis are emission spectrum and field size. The emission spectrum or *spectral power distribution* is the quality of a radiant energy source as measured by relative intensities plotted at various wavelengths (Fig 7–1). The *field size* of a light source is the area that can

TABLE 7-1.—LIGHT SOURCES USED IN CLINICAL PRACTICE

LIGHT SOURCE	EMISSION SPECTRUM DOSE (UVB)	ERYTHEMA TEST DOSE (UVA)	PHOTO PATCH	ADVANTAGES	DISADVANTAGES	MANUFACTURER	COST
Gas discharge arcs							
Low-pressure mercury cold quartz lamps	Discontinuous, predominantly 253.7 nm	30 sec at 25 cm	Not suitable	Cannot produce 2+ erythema, germicidal	3-minute warm-up	RA Fischer	$750–1,500
High-pressure mercury hot quartz lamp	Discontinuous, with peaks at 254,263,297,303, 365,405,440	10–30 mJ/sq cm; 30–60 sec at 45 cm; glass filters	0.5–1.5 J/sq cm; 7–20 min at 45 cm using window	Relatively inexpensive, intense UVB	3-minute warm-up; source for both therapy and diagnosis. Medium field size.	Hanovia, Sperti	$100–1,500
Medium-pressure metal halide	Continuous spectrum, 295–420 nm (4 mW/sq cm)	10–40 secs at 10 cm using special filter	30–90 secs at 40 cm	High-intensity UVA/SUP	2-minute warm-up; medium field size; bulb replacement at 1,000 hours; heat production; moderately expensive	UVATEC, NBL	$1,300–8,000

Lamp type	Spectral output	Dose	Treatment time	Advantages	Disadvantages	Manufacturers	Cost
Wood's lamp with nickel oxide filter	340–450 nm	Not suitable	5–10 min at 15 cm	Fluorescence test	Not suitable for phototherapy	Ultraviolet Products	$25–30
Fluorescent lamps							
UVB—Sunlamp	Continuous, 270–390 nm, peak 313 nm	10–30 mJ/sq cm = 60–120 sec at 25 cm, 30 min at 25 cm	Not suitable	Large field size when mounted in banks	Lamp output degrades with use, 70% at 500 hrs	Westinghouse	Tubes: $25–35 Cabinets: $2,000–10,000
Intermediate UVA/UVB	Continuous, 300–400 nm	——	——	Immediate warm-up time	High cost for cabinets and bulb replacement	Klafs Metec® Helarium, Dermacontrol	
UVA–black light	Continuous, 310–450 nm, peak 365 nm	——	5–30 min at 25 cm	Excellent source for phototesting	Energy per unit area less than mercury lamps	GE, Nat. Biol, Philips	$25–40/tube
Visible— "special blue daylight," etc.	Continuous 400–700 nm	——	——	Range of spectral distribution; Variety of purposes	Long treatment times; Multiple ballasts and cabinet construction result in heat production	Sylvania, Westinghouse	

SPECTRAL DISTRIBUTION COMPARISON

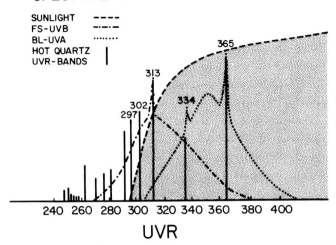

UVR

Fig 7–1.—By plotting the relative intensity against wavelength, qualitative differences between sunlight, hot quartz, and fluorescent lamps can be visualized. Since certain wavelengths of radiation are more efficient in producing certain photobiologic events, care must be taken to match the proper light source with the desired result.

be treated with a biologically effective dose of radiation in a reasonable period of time.

COMPARISON OF RADIANT LIGHT SOURCES[3, 12, 14]

Three major types of radiant light sources (see Table 7–1) are used in phototherapy apparatus available to the practicing dermatologist (and physiotherapist): the hot quartz (high-pressure mercury vapor) lamp; the metal halide lamp; and a variety of fluorescent bulbs. Each light source has its advantages, disadvantages, and clinical uses.

The medium- and high-pressure mercury vapor lamps have been used since the days of Goeckerman. When mercury vapor, enclosed in a quartz glass envelope, is ignited with an electric discharge arc, a characteristic series of discontinuous ultraviolet light wavelengths is produced (predominantly shorter wavelengths). As the lamp heats up, increasing pressure, a greater percentage of mid- and long-wave ultraviolet light is produced with correspondingly less UVC radiation produced. These lamps can be used for a variety of purposes: with a Wood's filter for fluorescent diagnosis, with a glass filter in photo patch testing, and in psoriasis phototherapy.

Owing to their moderate-to-small field size (intensity varies approximately inversely with the square of the distance between the light source and the target), hot quartz lamps usually are used to treat limited psoriatic disease (palms, soles, elbows, knees, etc.). However, because of their portability, they can be used for bedridden patients with generalized psoriasis by treating the patient in four to six segments. Although an intense source of UVB and relatively inexpensive, hot quartz lamps are today less popular owing to their field size, heat production, need for ventilation (ozone is initially produced when lamp is ignited), 3-minute lamp warm-up and required cooling-off period between treatments (if the lamp is extinguished). A typical hot quartz lamp is shown in Figure 7–2.

A recent entry on the market, metal halide lamps[24] are similar to mercury vapor lamps, except that with the addition of metal halide vapor and other gases, a continuous band of ultraviolet light wavelengths is produced. These units can be designed to deliver UVB or UVA radiation with internal or external filters. Despite their expense and excessive heat production, these lamps have the advantage of delivering more intense UVA (with appropriate UVB filters) than can be obtained from hot quartz lamps. Thus

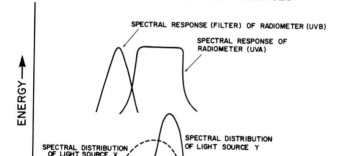

Fig 7–2.—The spectral response of the radiometer and the spectral distribution of the light source must be known and matched in any phototherapy system. Although the energy output of hypothetical UVA sources X and Y may be similar as measured by the same UVA (broadband filter) radiometer, their spectral distribution will likely produce different photobiologic effects. In this hypothetical example, a UVB radiometer would show the differences between these two light sources, but would not be measuring the bulk of the energy produced by the lamps.

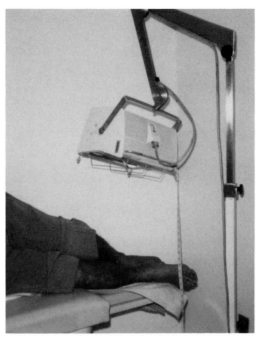

Fig 7–3.—A hot quartz lamp can deliver high-intensity UVB to a relatively small field and can be used for either adjunctive or primary phototherapy as well as skin testing.

they can be used for Goeckerman, PUVA, or the combination UVA/UVB selective ultraviolet light phototherapy (SUP) protocols popular in Europe. It may be a superior lamp for photo patch testing as well. A group of metal halide lamps may be mounted together to increase the treatment field size, as shown in Figure 7–3.

The source most suitable for psoriasis phototherapy is the fluorescent lamp. These lamps consist of a low-pressure mercury discharge arc whose 254-nm radiation excites a variety of phosphors coating the inside of a glass envelope tube, producing a continuous band of longer wavelengths. Depending on the phosphor and manufacturing process, a range of spectral distributions can be produced. The size (length and width), wattage, and other engineering factors (such as the presence of an internal reflecting coating) dictate the intensity of these lamps.

Morison and Pike[22] recently published careful spectral distribution measurement data on commonly used fluorescent ultraviolet light sources. Lamps used in the Goeckerman and outpatient psoriasis UVB phototherapy protocols include the Westinghouse FS series of lamps (in 2-, 4- and

6-foot sizes), whose output is approximately 60% UVB or shorter wavelengths and 40% UVA. On the other hand, typical UVA lamps produced for use in psoralen photochemotherapy by GTE, Sylvania, and National Biologic Corporation produced less than 3% UVB and 97% UVA, with around 20% of the radiation in the 320–340 nm range necessary to activate psoralens. Interestingly, other black lights designed for nonmedical purposes produce up to 99% UVA, but deliver virtually no 320–340 nm radiation and would therefore be inappropriate as a PUVA lamp.

The most recent addition to the list of ultraviolet fluorescent lamps is that produced by the Klafs Sunlight Corporation. This 100 watt Metec® Helarium bulb produces around 8% UVB and 92% UVA, of which approximately 30% is between 320–340 nm.[22] This lamp has been promoted as a combination UVA/UVB selective ultraviolet light phototherapy (SUP) source which can improve psoriasis with little to no erythema. It may also prove to be an excellent PUVA lamp (although its safety and efficacy needs further testing).

A bank of fluorescent lamps has the advantage of a relatively large field size, an immediate warm-up time, and relatively less heat production. Unfortunately, fluorescent lamp ultraviolet light output (and spectral distribution) degrades with time (70–80% of original output in 500 hours use) and it is usually recommended they be replaced after 1,000 hours of use. Lastly, multiple lamps and ballasts in an enclosed cabinet system often result in excessive heat production, even though individual fluorescent lamps put out very little heat.

EVALUATION OF RADIATION SOURCES[16]

Medical practice factors that affect the choice of phototherapy apparatus to be purchased include the estimated frequency and type of medical use; space, ventilation, and electrical requirements of the potential equipment location; and proposed budget and personnel. Equipment a dermatologist might recommend for home use will obviously differ in cost, size, and output from that to be used by a busy hospital service. Palmar, plantar, nail, and other localized forms of psoriasis are best treated with a hot quartz or metal halide UVB source or a well-designed fluorescent UVA source for PUVA. Generalized plaque or guttate psoriasis is usually best handled with fluorescent cabinets or panels. A typical hospital photomedicine unit should have at least one portable hot quartz (see Fig 7–2) or metal halide system (see Fig 7–3), and one combination UVA/UVB cabinet (Fig 7–4). A small, 8-to-16 bulb UVB phototherapy cabinet (Fig 7–5) is probably suffi-

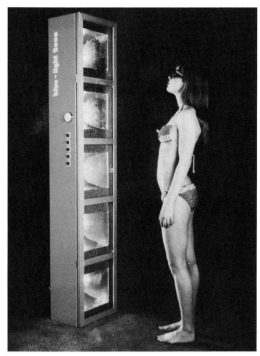

Fig 7–4.—Although comparatively expensive, metal halide lamp systems have the advantage over hot quartz lamps of providing a continuous UVB-UVA spectrum.

cient for most office practices. An example of a fluorescent hand and foot unit is shown in Figure 7–6.

Trying to compare the wide variety of phototherapeutic apparatus is like discussing automobile preferences. Some prefer expensive "European" models despite problems with long-term maintenance, while other physicians prefer the price of the small, simple, and efficient "Ford" over a "Cadillac" despite the latter's luxury, size, appearance, and electronic computer controls. A list of manufacturers who distribute phototherapy products in the U.S. can be found in Table 7–2. The features of a wide variety of products should be compared and scrutinized carefully before purchasing any of these products. Certain features (analogous to automobiles) are mandated by government regulations as specified by the Bureau of Radiological Health of the FDA.[1]

Features important to compare include technical features, safety/comfort features, size and appearance, flexibility, and cost (initial and maintenance/replacement). Technical features[25] include the type, size, number, and

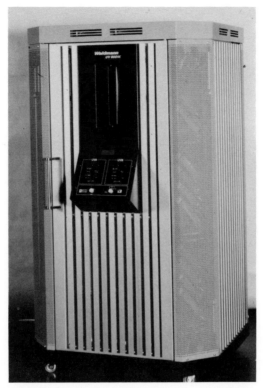

Fig 7–5.—A busy practice may require a unit that can deliver either UVB phototherapy or PUVA.

configuration of light sources; field size, lamp life, and warm-up time; dosimetry control including type, spectral response, and position on the radiometer (if included in the phototherapy system); and lastly, irradiance measurements (i.e., typical MED or MPD times). For example, a large practice with a number of severe psoriatics or a large population of more darkly pigmented psoriatics might require a unit with a greater number of bulbs and increased intensity in order to keep treatment times at a minimum. Folding cabinets may be built or purchased to conform to a small office.[27]

Safety/comfort features include shielding for staff, heat production/ventilation, handrails, protection from bulb breakage, windows for direct patient visualization, and timers, automatic shutoffs, and other fail-safe features of dosimetry control. Figure 7–5 shows a typical high intensity UVB fluorescent cabinet complete with windows, handrails, bulb protective screen, timers, and dosimetry control. Since the most common litigation

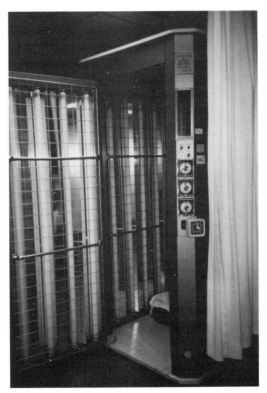

Fig 7–6.—Most office practices will only require a UVB unit. An 8- to 16-bulb unit is likely sufficient for most patients and the practice should compare prices of individual units with their individual features.

brought against dermatologists involves dosimetry error and ultraviolet light burns, this latter safety feature deserves special consideration. It must be pointed out, however, that very conscientious and carefully trained personnel are far more important than the most sophisticated (and expensive) dosimetry control system.

Open phototherapy cabinets are cooler in operation than closed systems, unless equipped with a very powerful heat exhaust system. Since closed systems may operate at approximately 20–25 F greater than the ambient temperature outside of the box, long treatments may produce discomfort and possible cardiovascular stress even with adequate air conditioning.[8, 9] Unfortunately, open phototherapy systems require extra diligence on the part of staff as well as curtains and other shields to prevent untoward ultraviolet light exposure to personnel.

Protection from bulb breakage is usually accomplished in two ways.

TABLE 7–2.—REPRESENTATIVE MANUFACTURERS OF PHOTOTHERAPY EQUIPMENT
(NOT INCLUSIVE)

MANUFACTURER	TYPE	MANUFACTURER	TYPE
Fluorescent UVR Systems		*Mercury Vapor & Woods Light Sources*	
DermaControl, Inc.	UVB, UVA, home	Burdick Corp.	parts only
14806 Drexel Ave.		Bay Shore, NY 11706	
Dolton, IL 60419		Milton, WI 53563	
(312) 841–8050		Conrad-Hanovia	UVB
Daavlin Company	UVB, UVA	100 Chestnut Street	
P.O. Box 626		Newark, NJ 07105	
Bryan, Ohio 43506		General Theraphysical (Hanau)	UVB
(419) 636–6304		2018 Washington	
Elder Pharmaceuticals	UVB, UVA	St. Louis, MO 63103	
Bryan, Ohio 43506		(314) 231–9643	
1–800–537–4294 (toll-free)		RA Fischer	UVC, Woods
in OH call collect:		517 Commercial Street	
(419) 636–1168		Glendale, CA 91203	
Environmental Growth	UVB, UVA	(213) 241–1178	
P.O. Box 407		Saalmann-SUP-Lampen	UVB-A
Chagrin Falls, OH 44022		Werrestrasse 94	
(216) 247–5100		D-4900 Herford-05221/24862	
Klafs Sunlight Corp.	UVB-A, home	West Germany	
210 Campus Drive		Spectronics	UVB, Woods
Arlington Hgts., IL 60004		956 Brush Hollow	
National Biologic Corp.	UVB, UVA, home	Westbury, NY 11590	
6057 Mayfield Rd.	(also metal halide)	(516) 333–4840	
Cleveland, OH 44124		Sperti Sunlamp Division	UVB, home
North Penn Mfg. Co.	UVB, home	20 Kenton Lands Road	
1100 Adams Ave.		Erlanger, KY 41018	
Philadelphia, PA 19124		(606) 331–0800	
(215) 288–0805		UVATEC	Dermalight, UVB
Richmond Light Co.	UVB, home	8430 Santa Monica Blvd.	(metal halide)
6023 Newington Drive		Los Angeles, CA 90069	
Richmond, VA 23224		(213) 650–0081	
UltraDerm Systems	UVA, UVB, home	*Radiometers*	
Professional Arts Bldg.		EG & G Electro-optics	
5090 State Street		35 Congress St.	
Saginaw, MI 48603		Salem, MA 01970	
(517) 792–6100		(617) 745–3200	
Ultralite Enterprises, Inc.	UVA	Eppley	
277 Industrial Park Dr.		12 Sheffield Ave.	
Lawrenceville, GA 30245		Newport, RI 02840	
(404) 936–0594		(401) 847–1020	
Waldmann Elektromedizinische	UVB, UVA	International Light	
Gerate		Dexter Industrial Green	
Postfach 1240		Newburyport, MA 01950	
D-7220 VS-Schwenningen		(617) 465–5923	
West Germany			

Acrylic or metal barriers and/or screening of various sizes, designed to prevent accidental direct contact of patients against the lamps, are often used in phototherapy cabinets. The ease with which these protective barriers can be removed is an important factor that determines downtime when lamp replacement is necessary. Plastic sleeves can be placed around the fluorescent tubes: for example, Mylar®, which blocks out stray UVB, around UVA lamps or ultraviolet light-translucent Teflon® FEP in UVB systems. Handrails can also guard against accidental bulb breakage that can result if patients lose their balance and fall into the fluorescent lamps.

Home phototherapy equipment,[17, 18, 21] which is found to be effective in certain cases of psoriasis and mycosis fungoides, requires very careful patient selection before any recommendations can be made. Apparatus ranges from very inexpensive hot quartz lamps, to moderately priced fluorescent panels, to more expensive but safer key-dependent enclosed systems designed to meet FDA specifications and generally modeled after the original Zimmerman cabinet.[28] The choice of which of these products should be prescribed is often influenced by which units are underwritten by medical insurance plans and/or a patient's financial status.

EQUIPMENT ACCESSORIES

Eye protection apparatus is absolutely necessary for patients (and staff) during treatment, and in the case of PUVA, up to 24 hours after the ingestion of psoralens to protect from direct sun or bright window exposure.[2, 10, 19, 23] Goggles, wraparound UV-opaque glasses, and coated lenses may be obtained from ultraviolet light equipment manufacturers or directly from companies listed in Table 7–3.

Templates needed to perform MED light dose titration may be made from opaque adhesive tape strips or can be obtained from: Higgins Die and Cutting, 49 D Street, South Boston, Massachusetts 02127 (specify 3¼ × 4-inch foil masks; $200/1,000 in 1984). Alternatively, reusable templates can be obtained from manufacturers such as Waldmann or Daavlin.

Radiometers are optional with some phototherapy equipment. They are essential for PUVA protocols and are helpful in UVB phototherapy when a patient transfers from one treatment center to another. They are also useful in determining when to change lamps and how an individual phototherapy unit compares to those discussed in the literature. It is likely that when a radiometer comes with the ultraviolet light equipment, it is the appropriately calibrated unit; however, care must be taken to purchase a radiometer with a sensor and filter system matched to the phototherapy equipment you are using. If a radiometer calibrated for UVB is used for a UVA system, differing results will be recorded, as illustrated in Figure 7–7. Also, radiometers must be recalibrated at least yearly to remain reliable. A variety of radiometers is available and can be obtained from the phototherapy equipment manufacturers or directly from the companies listed in Table 7–2.

Individual chemical dosimeters[7, 11, 15] (miniature radiometers) are being

TABLE 7–3.—PHOTOPROTECTIVE EYE APPARATUS

PRODUCT NAME	MANUFACTURER	FEATURES
Goggles Worn During Treatment		
NOIRettes	Recreational Innovations Co. P.O. Box 159 South Lyon, Michigan 48178 (313) 769–5565	
Super Sunnies	Lucas Products Corp. Toledo, Ohio 43612	
Wraparound Glasses (UVA and UVB)		
NOIR	Recreational Innovations Co. P.O. Box 159 South Lyon, Michigan 48178 (313) 769–5565	Models 101 or 501: amber; Models 102 or 502: gray-green; worn over prescription frames; cost: $13.50 plus $2.10 shipping and handling
Blak-Ray	UVP, Inc. (formerly Ultraviolet Products, Inc.) 5100 Walnut Grove Avenue San Gabriel, California 91778 (213) 285–3123	Model: Contract Control Spectacles UVC-303: yellow tinted or clear; worn over prescription frames; cost: $6.00
Silver-Shield goggles	Dioptics Medical Products 15550 Rockfield Blvd., Suite C Irvine, California 92718 (714) 859–7111	Tinted brown or gray; cost: $5.50 + shipping
Clear UVA Blocking Lens		
UV 400 (Orcolite)	Dioptics Medical Products; order thru local optician (patient brochures available)	Clear or tinted; cost: approximately $10 more than ordinary prescription lenses; determined by optician
UV 400 clip-ons	Dioptics Medical Products; order through above address	Amber or gray tint; worn over prescription frames; cost: $18.00/ pair through dermatologist

developed that may be helpful in protecting staff and useful in developing patient protocols, particularly for home phototherapy. An integrating dose measuring device is presently available from the International Light Corporation for use with psoralens and sunlight that automatically takes into account cloud cover and time of day as it measures the total cumulative dose of UVA received from sunlight over a specific time. A patient can key in the specific dose of light in terms of energy he is to receive, and a timer goes off when the patient has received this dose of sunlight. Similar equipment could be designed for UVB protocols.

PERSPECTIVES

As new phototherapy protocols are developed, improvements in phototherapy equipment are likely. Individual dosimeter protocols, improve-

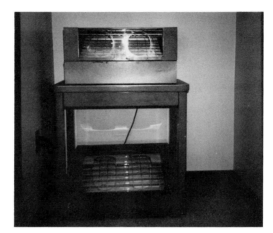

Fig 7–7.—A specialized hand and foot UVA unit is good for treating disabling psoriasis of the palms and/or soles without the risks of treatment to the rest of the body.

ments in dosimetry controls, and improved design in radiometers and light sources are but a few examples of changes we will undoubtedly see over the next few years. Despite this, there is presently an abundance of excellent phototherapy apparatus available for the treatment of psoriasis. Hopefully, the points made in this chapter will assist the practitioner in either purchasing or recommending specific equipment for their individual patient needs.

REFERENCES

1. Devices used as a radiation source (in combination with psoralen drug) in the photochemotherapy for psoriasis. *Federal Register* USDHEW, February, 1980.
2. Editorial: Current status of oral PUVA therapy for psoriasis. *J. Am. Acad. Dermatol.* 1:106–117, 1979.
3. Environmental Health Criteria 14: Ultraviolet radiation. Geneva: United Nations Environmental Health Organization, World Health Organization, and International Radiation Protection Association, Finland, 1979.
4. Aeling J.L., Nuss D.D.: Outpatient modified Goeckerman regimen. *J. Assoc. Military Dermatol.* 3:10–12, 1977.
5. Beckett R.H.: *Modern Actinotherapy.* London: William Heinemann Medical Books, 1955, pp. 1–63.
6. Bickford F.D.: Risks associated with use of UV-A irradiators being used in treating psoriasis and other conditions. *Lighting Design and Application*, March, 1979, pp. 56–58.
7. Brauer H.-D., Schmidt R.: A new reusable chemical actinometer for UV irradiation in the 248–334 nm range. *Photochem. Photobiol.* 37(5):587–591, 1983.
8. Chappe S.G., Roegnigk H.H., Miller A.J., et al.: The effect of photochemotherapy on the cardiovascular system. *J. Am. Acad. Dermatol.* 4:561–565, 1981.
9. Ciafone R.A., Rhodes A.R., Audley M., et al.: The cardiovascular stress of photochemotherapy (PUVA). *J. Am. Acad. Dermatol.* 3:499–505, 1980.

10. Davey J.B., Diffey B.L., Miller J.A.: Eye protection in psoralen photochemotherapy. *Br. J. Dermatol.* 104:295–300, 1981.
11. Fanselow D.L., et al.: Reusable ultraviolet monitors: Design, characteristics, and efficacy. *J. Am. Acad. Dermatol.* 9:714–723, 1983.
12. Harbes L.C., Bickers D., Epstein J.H.: Light sources used in photopatch testing, in Fitzpatrick T. (ed.): *Sunlight and Man: Normal and Abnormal Photobiologic Responses.* Tokyo, University of Tokyo Press, 1974, pp. 559–574.
13. Fitzpatrick T.B., Haynes H., Parrish J.A.: Is UVA safe? *Dermatologic Capsule and Comment* 2:4–8, 1980.
14. Harber L.C., Bickers D.R.: *Photosensitivity Diseases: Principles of Diagnosis and Treatment.* Philadelphia, W.B. Saunders Co., 1981.
15. Holman C.D.J., et al.: Ultraviolet irradiation of human body sites in relation to occupation and outdoor activity: Field studies using personal UVR dosimeters. *Clin. Exper. Dermatol.* 8:269–277, 1983.
16. Horwitz S.N., Frost P.: A phototherapy cabinet for ultraviolet radiation therapy. *Arch. Dermatol.* 117:469–473, 1981.
17. Jordan W.P., Clarke A.M., Hale R.K.: Long-term modified Goeckerman regimen for psoriasis using an ultraviolet B light source in the home. *J. Am. Acad. Dermatol.* 4:584–591, 1981.
18. Larko O., Swanbeck G.: Home solarium treatment of psoriasis. *Br. J. Dermatol.* 101:13–16, 1979.
19. Lerman S., Megaw J., Willis I.: Potential ocular complications from PUVA therapy and their prevention. *J. Invest. Dermatol.* 74:197–199, 1980.
20. Magnus I.A.: *Dermatologic Photobiology.* London, Blackwell Scientific Publications, 1976, pp. 41–53.
21. Milstein H.J., Vonderheid E.C., Van Scott E.J., et al.: Home ultraviolet phototherapy for early mycosis fungoides: Preliminary observations. *J. Am. Acad. Dermatol.* 6:355–362, 1982.
22. Morison W.L., Pike R.A.: Spectral power distributions of radiation sources used in phototherapy and photochemotherapy. *J. Am. Acad. Dermatol.* 10:64–68, 1984.
23. Morison W.L., Strickland P.T.: Environmental UVA radiation and eye protection during PUVA therapy. *J. Am. Acad. Dermatol.* 9:522–525, 1983.
24. Mutzhas M.F., Holze E., Hofmann C., et al.: A new apparatus with high radiation energy between 320–460 nm: Physical description and dermatological applications. *J. Invest. Dermatol.* 76:42–47, 1981.
25. Nachtwey D.S., Rundel R.D.: A photobiological evaluation of tanning booths. *Science* 211:405–407, 1981.
26. Parrish J., Anderson R., Urbach F., et al.: UVA: Biological effects of ultraviolet radiation with emphasis on human responses to long-wave ultraviolet, in Sources of UVA. New York, Plenum Press, 1978, pp. 7–34.
27. Witten V.H.: A folding ultraviolet light box. *Arch. Dermatol.* 107:716, 1973.
28. Zimmerman M.C.: Ultraviolet light therapy: Utilization of tubular fluorescent lamps in a cabinet for generalized simultaneous irradiation. *Arch. Dermatol.* 78:646–652, 1958.

8 / Tar and Ultraviolet Therapy

STEPHEN HORWITZ, M.D.

ONE CLASSIC METHOD for treating severe psoriasis consists of the application of a tar preparation followed by exposure to gradually increasing doses of ultraviolet-B (UVB) radiation (UVBR). Since the introduction of Goeckerman's original regimen in 1925, many modifications have been proposed. In any of its many forms, the use of UVB radiation in conjunction with topical therapies has remained the mainstay of psoriasis therapy for patients with extensive, severe psoriasis.

PATIENT SELECTION

Because of its record of efficacy and safety, phototherapy is one treatment of choice for patients who have extensive plaque psoriasis. Extensive psoriasis may be arbitrarily defined as involvement of greater than 20% of the body surface. Phototherapy occasionally may be used for patients with less extensive psoriasis that is refractory to adequate courses of other conventional therapies (e.g., topical or intralesional corticosteroids, anthralin, or tar). Phototherapy is also useful for pustular and erythrodermic psoriasis, but it must be administered cautiously to avoid exacerbation of the disease. Approximately 10% of patients do not respond to PUVA phototherapy, but their lesions may clear with a tar-UVBR phototherapy regimen.

ADMINISTRATION OF UVB RADIATION

The most difficult and controversial part of treatment is administering UVB radiation effectively. Much of the difficulty arises because the equipment used to deliver and measure UVB radiation is not standardized. The most convenient measure of light dose is time; however, because of the differences in light sources (type of lamp; whether hot quartz or fluorescent; number, arrangement, and age of bulbs), the amount of UVB energy delivered per unit of time is highly variable. It is therefore impossible to give specific recommendations for treatment times for UVB radiation. In addition, the dose of UVB must be tailored individually for each patient because of differences in sensitivity. The initial dose of UVB can either be estimated from the patient's previous sunburn history or determined by exposure to graduated doses of UVB radiation to identify the MED.

A system of skin typing based on the patient's previous sunburn history has been advocated (Table 8–1). To determine the skin type by this method, the patient's skin response to the initial midday summer sun exposure is ascertained and assigned a number from I to IV (most sun-sensitive to least). In theory, each skin type should correspond to a discrete, narrow range of MEDs and an appropriate dose of UVB. In this author's experience, however, there may be considerable overlap of MEDs among patients of different skin types,[1] so that the skin type method is not an accurate guide to selecting the initial UVBR dose.

The Minimal Erythema Dose (MED)

The only accurate method for identifying the proper initial UVB dose is to determine the MED for each patient before beginning therapy. In this way, the initial dose of UVB radiation will not be so excessive as to produce a burn nor will it be so low as to be less than the threshold dose necessary to be effective in clearing the psoriatic plaques.

The MED is determined by exposing small test squares of skin to gradually increasing amounts of UVB radiation to identify the lowest dose that

TABLE 8–1.—EXPOSURE GUIDE FOR DETERMINING THE MINIMAL
ERYTHEMA DOSE

SKIN TYPE	DESCRIPTION	EXPOSURE RANGE*
I	Always burns, never tans	30, 60, 90, 120, 240 (sec)
II	Always burns, sometimes tans	
III	Sometimes burns, always tans	1, 2, 3, 4, 5, 6 (min)
IV	Never burns, always tans	

*These numbers are meant only to serve as a guideline for the phototherapy cabinet described by Horwitz and Frost.[2] Other types of UV equipment will have significantly different times for MEDs.

produces barely perceptible erythema 24 hours after exposure. For best results, the UVBR exposure is performed with the same light source and topical medications that will be used for therapy. A template made of felt, cardboard, or other opaque material into which six 1-cm squares have been cut is applied to the skin. The exposed skin outside of the template is covered with an opaque cloth, leaving only the skin within the fenestrations of the template exposed. The site for locating the template, usually on the torso, is selected according to the amount and distribution of tan and psoriasis on the body. If the amount of tan is the same for all parts of the body, the template can be located anywhere there is an area free of psoriasis. On the other hand, when the patient has some areas that are tan and some areas that have had no sunlight (for example, bathing trunk area and breasts), the MED should be performed on an area of skin, usually the back, in which the degree of tanning is intermediate between the covered areas, such as the buttocks, and the most heavily tanned area, such as the upper back.

The duration of light exposure required to produce a MED varies among light sources because there is no uniformity in construction of UVB cabinets and no standard method for measuring UVB radiation levels. The MED determination functions as a simple biologic dosimeter by integrating the light box design and the skin sensitivity into one measurement. For any given light cabinet, the proper dosage range of UVB exposures for MED testing can best be determined by measuring the MEDs of several patients with varying degrees of pigmentation, starting at low exposures and gradually increasing the exposure time.

Although skin typing is not sufficient for determining the initial treatment dose, it may be a useful guide to the exposure range for accurately determining the MED. For example, in the light cabinet designed by the author,[2] exposures of 30, 60, 90, 120, 180, and 240 seconds are used for patients with skin types I and II. For patients with skin types III and IV, exposure intervals of 1, 2, 3, 4, 5, and 6 minutes may be more likely to identify the MED (see Table 8–1).

The MED exposure sites are read 24 hours after the exposure and the MED is defined as the lowest dose of UVB radiation that will produce erythema filling the square. The ambient lighting should be standardized when interpreting MED test results since variations in the ambient light can influence the color of the skin. Once the MED has been determined, the treatment regimen may begin.

TREATMENT REGIMENS FOR CLEARING PSORIASIS

Two dosage regimens have been advocated for administering UVB radiation: erythemogenic and suberythemogenic. The two regimens have been shown, in controlled studies, to be equally effective in clearing psoriasis with the same number of UVBR treatments.[1, 3–5]

Erythemogenic Dosage Schedule[6–9]

When erythemogenic doses of UVB radiation are administered, the amount of UVB that can be administered is limited by the development of erythema of normal-appearing skin. Numerous methods have been proposed for selecting the daily dose of UVB. The easiest method is to start with 50%–100% of the MED for the first dose. Subsequent doses of UVBR are increased by a fixed percentage (15%–25%) of the previous day's dose in order to maintain mild, nontender erythema of the normal-appearing skin when examined 24 hours later. If tender erythema is present, the treatments should be withheld until the erythema subsides.

Suberythemogenic Dosage Schedule

In 1978, Frost, et al. introduced an alternative method of administering the proper dose of UVBR.[1] It is designed to use the lowest dose of UVB radiation commensurate with improvement. The theory behind this regimen is that as long as there is improvement in the psoriatic plaques, there is no need to increase the dose of UVB. Improvement is measured by means of a severity score of representative psoriatic plaques.

The initial dose of UVB is 50% of the MED. Subsequent doses are determined by assessing the improvement of four representative psoriatic plaques. Improvement is defined as a three-point decrease in the total severity score over a two-day period.

SEVERITY SCORE.—The total severity score is the sum of the scores for erythema, scaling, and thickness, each rated on a 0–6 scale for each of four representative psoriatic plaques that are evaluated daily prior to UVB treatment (Table 8–2). The maximum severity score is 72 (4 plaques × maximum score of 6 × 3 parameters). The plaques selected for evaluation should be on the trunk or on the extremities, proximal to the elbows and

TABLE 8–2.—SCORING SYSTEM FOR ERYTHEMA,
SCALING AND THICKNESS

Erythema
    0—Absence of color change (normal skin)
    1—Trace of pink (barely perceptible)
    2—Pink
    3—Dark pink
    4—Scarlet (red)
    5—Crimson (dark red)
    6—Maroon or purple-red
Scaling
    0—Absence of visible scale (normal skin)
    1—Trace; few, small, thin scales
    2—Mild; small, discrete scales
    3—Mild to moderate; mainly small, thin scales, some
       thick scales present
    4—Moderate; combined thick and thin scales, equally
       distributed
    5—Moderate to severe; mainly large, thick scales,
       some areas with thin scales
    6—Severe; ostraceous scaling; thick, white-silvery,
       opaque scales covering entire lesion
Thickness
    0—Nonpalpable
    1—Trace; barely perceptible with touch, not with
       vision
    2—Mild; definitely perceptible with touch, not with
       vision
    3—Mild to moderate; perceptible with touch and
       vision
    4—Moderate; definite elevation
    5—Moderate to severe; plateau-like elevation of lesions
       (less than 2 mm)
    6—Severe; plateau-like elevation of lesions (greater
       than 2 mm)

knees. The reason for excluding the plaques on the elbows, knees, and distal extremities is that psoriasis on these anatomical areas typically clears more slowly even with additional UVB treatment. Evaluating plaques from these areas results in use of higher doses of UVB than necessary to clear the majority of the psoriatic plaques, without enhancing the clearing of the more resistant plaques.

CALCULATING THE DAILY UVB DOSE.—Each day's total severity score is compared with the previous two days' severity scores. If there has been a decrease of three or more points, then the dose of UVB remains the same. If there has not been a three-point decrease in severity score, then the dose of radiation is increased. A sample treatment record is shown in Figure 8–1.

				DERMATOLOGY PHOTOTHERAPY TREATMENT			
				DOCTOR _____			
				DIAGNOSIS _____			
				TREATMENT _____			
				SKIN TYPE _____			
				MEDICATIONS _____			
DATE	TX #	INTENSITY	TODAY JOULE/cm²	TOTAL DOSE	CUMULATIVE TIME/MIN	TODAY mg 8 MOP	PHYSICIAN'S SIGNATURE

DERMATOLOGY PHOTOTHERAPY TREATMENT

Fig 8–1.—Example of a PUVA, UVB, tar or anthralin record sheet used in a treatment center.

DOSAGE INCREMENTS.—Sample dosage increments are presented in Table 8–3. The dosage increments are gradually increased as the daily dose increases: the smallest increments occur at the lowest treatment times and, as the treatment time becomes longer, the increment becomes greater. This is done to compensate for tanning, which occurs as a result of the treatment. Although the regimen is designed to clear psoriasis without producing erythema of uninvolved skin, UVB-induced erythema may occasionally occur if the dose is increased when the patient has not improved. Ad-

TABLE 8–3.—TABLE FOR DETERMINING
DOSAGE INCREMENT*

PREVIOUS TREATMENT DOSE		INCREMENT†
Time (min)	mJ	Sec (mJ)
0–2	0–12	15 (1.5)
2–5	12–30	30 (3.0)
5–10	30–60	60 (6.0)
>10	>60	120 (12.0)

*The dosage increment is varied according to the duration of the previous treatment dose. This table applies to patients receiving treatments at least twice a week.

†The increment values for time listed in this table apply only to the light cabinet designed by the author[2] and are based on multiples of 1.5 mJ of energy. For other light cabinets, the exposure times that correspond to the energy levels can be calculated from the following formula:

$$\text{Time (sec)} = \frac{\text{Energy (J/sq cm)}}{\text{Meter Reading (W/sq cm)}}$$

e.g., 15 seconds of exposure equals 0.0015 J/sq cm when the meter reading is 0.00015 W/sq cm.

justments in the dosage schedule may then be necessary. If nontender erythema is present, then the previous day's dose is repeated regardless of the severity score. If tender erythema is present 24 hours after the treatment, then no treatment is given that day.

ADVANTAGES.—There are a number of advantages of the suberythemogenic treatment regimen:

1. The severity score system provides a quantitive method by which the response of the psoriasis to the therapy can easily be followed. (This applies whether erythemogenic or suberythemogenic treatment schedules are used.)

2. The dose of UVB is tailored to suit each patient. The lowest dose of UVB that clears the psoriatic plaques is used, and UVB-induced burns, which are painful and potentially harmful, are avoided.

3. Lower cumulative doses of UVB are safer.

4. The dosage increment system takes the guesswork out of administering the therapy and can be administered safely by a trained technician.

SCHEDULE OF UVB TREATMENTS

Besides the dosage of UVBR, the two factors that are most important for clearing of psoriasis are the total number of treatments and the frequency with which those treatments are administered. On average, 20–30 UVB treatments are necessary to clear psoriasis. The average number of treatments to clear is the same whether the treatments are given three, five, or seven days a week; however, patients who receive the treatments less than three times a week usually do much more poorly than patients receiving treatments three or more times a week. This point cannot be overemphasized since treatments given too infrequently or discontinued prematurely are the most common causes of treatment failure and early relapse after treatment.

TOPICAL MEDICATIONS

The standard Goeckerman regimen consists of UVB radiation administered in conjunction with coal tar applied at bedtime and emollients applied to the skin during the day. Crude coal tar ointment in concentrations ranging from 1%–5% in petrolatum was, until recently, the standard formulation. The disadvantages of these ointments include staining of skin, clothes, and linens; an objectionable odor; and folliculitis. For these reasons, this treatment was generally reserved for hospitalized patients. Outpatient therapy has become more practical with the introduction of tar gel formulations (Table 8–4). These contain distillates of crude coal tar in more cosmetically acceptable gel bases. The tar gels can be rubbed into the skin better than the tar ointments, leaving less on the surface to stain bedclothes and linens. They are also perfumed to conceal the smell, and they are more easily washed off with soap and water. These features improve patient acceptability and compliance and have made home therapy easier. Most important, the tar gels have been shown to be as effective as the coal tar ointments in clearing psoriasis.[10]

If coal tar ointment is used, a 1% concentration is as effective as a 5% or 25% concentration. Coal tar penetrates the stratum corneum readily and

TABLE 8–4.—TAR PREPARATIONS

PRODUCT	COMPOSITION
Baker's P and S Plus Tar Gel	Coal tar solution (8%)* and salicylic acid (2%) in a moisturizing gel (6% alcohol)
Estar Gel	Biologically equivalent to 5% coal tar U.S.P. contained in a hydroalcoholic gel (29% alcohol)
Psorigel	7.5% coal tar solution and 33% alcohol
T-Derm	5% tar body oil in its oil base

*Equivalent to 1.6% crude coal tar.

need only be applied for two hours a day, although overnight application may be more convenient.[8] The tar products do not need to be on the skin at the time of UVB exposure, since there is no photointeraction between coal tar and UVB radiation.[11]

The role of tar in the Goeckerman regimen has recently been questioned. In 1980, LeVine, et al. compared the effectiveness of a tar gel, a coal tar ointment in petrolatum, and plain petrolatum in combination with erythemogenic UVB radiation for clearing psoriasis.[13] Their findings were that petrolatum applied immediately prior to the UVB exposure was as effective as the tar preparations. They hypothesized that the application of the ointment made the psoriatic scales more transparent, thereby decreasing reflection and scatter of UVB radiation and enhancing penetration.[13]

Lowe, et al. demonstrated that with suberythemogenic doses of UVBR, coal tar preparations are superior to emollient bases alone for clearing psoriasis, whereas with erythemogenic doses of UVBR, tar preparations were equivalent to emollients.[3] In both studies, as in our study,[1] UVBR alone did not completely clear psoriasis.

ADJUNCTIVE THERAPY

Keratolytics

The thick, silvery scale on psoriatic plaques can reduce the effectiveness of the UVB radiation. Petrolatum or a similar emollient applied immediately prior to UVB exposure can make the scale transparent, but it leaves a greasy residue on the skin. Hydration of the stratum corneum by applying water to the scaly plaques before the treatment will make the scales transparent but may be impractical. Removal of excess scale during the first week of phototherapy by chemical methods (salicylic acid, 2–10% in ointment base) or mechanical methods (abrasive sponge) may be useful. Keratolytics are discussed in detail in Chapter 5.

Anthralin

Anthralin, in cream or ointment base, may be applied to resistant plaques, but it has not been shown to reduce the number of UVB treatments needed to clear psoriasis. Conventional overnight anthralin therapy is not well tolerated in outpatient usage because it irritates normal skin and stains skin and clothing; however, short-contact anthralin therapy is often tolerated. Anthralin therapy is discussed more fully in Chapter 6.

Corticosteroids

Topically applied corticosteroids are the most commonly used adjuncts to phototherapy. In an uncontrolled study, 0.1% triamcinolone cream under occlusion reduced the number of UVB treatments needed to achieve clearing.[14] In controlled prospective studies, however, topical corticosteroids did not reduce the number of treatments required to clear the psoriasis, the cumulative dose of UVB, or the frequency of UVB radiation burns.[15, 16] More important, the addition of a topically applied corticosteroid leads to earlier relapse of disease.[17, 18] They should not be used in patients with extensive psoriasis except for very brief periods to treat skin sites not accessible to UVB radiation, such as the scalp, groin, and skin folds.

Methotrexate

Methotrexate is effective for controlling severe psoriasis. To be effective when used alone, it requires chronic administration, which may produce hepatotoxicty. In one study, patients with very resistant psoriasis were successfully treated with methotrexate alone weekly for three weeks then combined with UVBR phototherapy, twice weekly, for an additional four weeks, for a total of seven doses. Remission times were not reported.[19]

PUVA

Combining UVB and PUVA phototherapy has been reported to reduce the total number of UVB treatments and the total dose of ultraviolet-A required to clear psoriasis.[20, 21]

ADVERSE REACTIONS

UVB-Related

SUNBURN.—The most frequent adverse effect of phototherapy is the development of a UVB-induced sunburn. It may occur at any time during the course of therapy and usually is the result of exceeding the patient's MED. Other causes of erythema must be considered. It is important to obtain a complete drug history before starting treatment, since many medications can interact with UVB radiation, producing a phototoxic reaction that could be mistaken for an exacerbation of psoriasis. The most commonly implicated drugs are diuretics (particularly thiazide type), oral hypoglycemic agents, antibiotics (sulfonamides), antiarrhythmic agents (particularly quinidine), soporifics, and antianxiety agents. Topical medications, especially sunscreening agents, may occasionally result in a contact photodermatitis. Patients must be cautioned against exposure to natural sunlight without adequate protection, since this could result in unintentional overexposure to UVB radiation. A careful history will eliminate patients with known photosensitivity diseases, such as lupus erythematosus, polymorphous light eruption, and porphyria cutanea tarda.

CONJUNCTIVITIS.—UVB-induced conjunctivitis is an acute, painful reaction to the exposure of unprotected eyes to UVB radiation. Patients should be required to wear protective glasses during treatment. Almost all commercially available glass and plastic lenses will absorb UVB radiation. Protective goggles made specifically for use with UVB therapy are available from several suppliers. Plastic eyecups used by swimmers are readily available in smoke tint or clear lenses and effectively filter UVB radiation. This type of eye covering is preferable to sunglasses since they fit firmly against the periorbital skin; sunglasses may allow stray UVB radiation to reach the eye. A quick office test can verify their effectiveness by placing the goggles or glasses between the sensor of the UVB photometer and the lighted bulbs; the reading should be zero.

The time course of the UVB-induced conjunctivitis is similar to that of UVB-induced erythema. Signs and symptoms of burning, tearing, and photophobia are present six hours after UVBR exposure and peak at about 24 hours. Symptoms begin to subside between 24 and 48 hours after exposure, and the patient is generally asymptomatic after 72 hours. This, of course, can vary with the amount of UVB exposure. Treatment is usually not necessary, but the patient should see an ophthalmologist since similar symptoms may be caused by infection or corneal abrasion. UVB-induced conjunctivitis occurs most often because patients remove the glasses during treatment to inspect their skin or to try to tan the skin that is normally protected by the goggles. Patients should be specifically cautioned against these violations.

MISCELLANEOUS SKIN REACTIONS.—Exposure to UVB radiation may precipitate a recurrence of herpes simplex labialis in susceptible patients.

If a patient has a history of herpes simplex labialis that recurs from sunlight exposure, it is helpful to apply a sunscreen to the lips and perioral skin.

About 10% of patients will experience a mild flare of psoriasis during the course of UVB treatment. This usually appears as small red macules and papules, often in sites that previously had no psoriasis. These are temporary and disappear with reassurance and continued therapy.

Areas of persistent scaling that fail to improve with therapy, particularly on the lower extremities and feet, may indicate concurrent dermatophyte infection. Skin scrapings for potassium hydroxide examination and fungal culture are helpful.

The effect of long-term UVB exposure that is of the greatest concern is the development of UVB-induced skin tumors. Recent retrospective reviews have failed to demonstrate an increased risk of skin cancer in psoriasis patients receiving phototherapy,[22-24] while another retrospective review suggested that there may be an increased risk of developing certain skin cancers.[25] However, these findings need to be confirmed by carefully controlled prospective studies.

Topical Therapy

Topically applied medications used in phototherapy are occasional sources of problems. Folliculitis can be minimized if coal tar ointments are applied to hair-bearing surfaces in the same direction as the hair grows. This theoretically minimizes forcing of tar into the hair follicles. The use of tar gels has largely eliminated this complication.

Unknown Causes

Pruritus is a frequent side effect of phototherapy. It is usually seen at the end of the first week of therapy and may persist until the psoriatic lesions have cleared. Although the true etiology of this complication is not known, it is suspected that dryness of the skin induced by both the UVB radiation and the tar gel preparations may be contributory. The alcohol in the gel base of the tar products may account for these effects. Liberal applications of bland emollients in the morning after showering and in the afternoon may be helpful. They may either be occlusive (e.g., mineral oil or petrolatum based) or water retentive (e.g., phospholipid-based), the latter being more cosmetically acceptable. Antihistaminic agents have rarely been helpful for this very distressing reaction.

A less frequent reaction of unknown etiology is the development of multiple verrucous papules. Histologically, these have the appearance of squamous papillomas. They do not show features of viral warts and we have been unable to identify wart antigen within these papules. (S. Horwitz, unpublished data). Liquid nitrogen briefly applied to the individual warts is a simple, effective treatment.

ASSESSMENT OF RESPONSE TO UVBR THERAPY

Improvement proceeds in an orderly fashion in most patients. The most notable change in the first week is a reduction in the amount of scale on the psoriatic plaque. Erythema and induration then decrease to the point that the plaques begin to break up into small papules by the end of the second week. At the same time, a clear halo may form around the psoriatic plaques. This is known as *Woronoff's ring*. The appearance of this ring usually indicates improvement of the psoriatic plaques.

TREATMENT FAILURES

The most difficult aspect of UVB phototherapy is evaluating the patient whose lesions do not clear with therapy. What is meant by "clear" must be defined: if a patient has not improved by at least 50% of his severity score at the end of 28 treatments, then he or she may be considered a treatment failure. However, since some patients require 40 or 42 treatments to clear, the patient should be encouraged to continue the therapy if there is some degree of improvement. Review what topical medications should be used at home, since patients often change their regimen without informing the physician. Check to see whether the patient has started using any new medications that may interfere with improvement in the psoriasis. Approximately 10% of patients with psoriasis will not clear with UVB phototherapy. For these patients, either adjunctive therapy or alternative forms of phototherapy, such as psoralen plus UVA phototherapy or systemic therapy, should be considered.

PATIENT EDUCATION

Proper education of the new patient is essential for successful phototherapy. Two aspects of the treatment program should be stressed at the onset

TABLE 8–5.—INSTRUCTION SHEET FOR PSORIASIS PATIENTS RECEIVING TAR AND ULTRAVIOLET THERAPY

You are receiving a sophisticated form of therapy for your psoriasis. This treatment requires your cooperation and attention to be a success. Please adhere to the following schedule.

1. At bedtime: (Tar Gel)	Bathe or shower with soap and water, if you wish. Apply tar to *entire* body including scalp (if involved). After 20 minutes you may apply a moisturizer, such as Complex 15, Panscol ointment, or petrolatum, to your skin.
2. Upon arising:	Bathe or shower with soap and water. Shampoo with tar shampoo.
3. Light treatment:	Do not apply any lotions or ointment within 4 hours prior to light treatment. If it is longer than 4 hours from the time of your bath or shower to your light treatment, you may apply a moisturizer.
4. After light treatment: (Moisturizer)	After your light treatment a moisturizer such as Complex 15 (cream or lotion), Panscol (cream or lotion), or Vaseline should be applied to your skin. This will help reduce dryness and itching of your skin. You should apply one of these at least 2 to 3 times daily.
IMPORTANT:	You should avoid excess sunlight exposure on the day of your light treatment, since this could result in a severe sunburn. Natural sunlight is most intense between 10:00 A.M. and 3:00 P.M. Be particularly careful if you are outdoors during these hours by wearing clothing and by applying sunscreen (SPF 15) on sun-exposed surfaces.

---

to insure compliance and to minimize patient dissatisfaction. First, the patient should be given an information sheet outlining the daily regimen of topical therapy and ultraviolet exposure (Table 8–5). This should be reviewed in detail with the patient. Second, the patient should be told that clearing of psoriasis requires an average of 20 to 30 treatments and that treatments should be given no less than three times a week. Last, the patient needs to be informed that the treatment will control, not cure, psoriasis and that the goal of therapy is to induce a remission that may last from weeks to years.[24] These points must be emphasized frequently during the course of therapy, otherwise the patient may have unreasonable expectations that can lead to frustration.

REFERENCES

1. Frost P., Horwitz S.N., Caputo R.V., Berger S.M.: Tar gel-phototherapy for psoriasis. *Arch. Dermatol.* 115:840–846, 1979.
2. Horwitz S., Frost P.: A phototherapy cabinet for treating psoriasis. *Arch. Dermatol.* 117:469–473, 1981.
3. Lowe N.J., Wortzman M.S., Breeding J., et al.: Coal tar phototherapy for psoriasis reevaluated: Erythemogenic versus suberythemogenic ultraviolet with a tar extract in oil and crude coal tar. *J. Am. Acad. Dermatol.* 8:781–789, 1982.
4. Eells L.D., Wolff J.M., Garloff J., et al.: Comparison of suberythemogenic and maximally aggressive ultraviolet B therapy for psoriasis. *J. Am. Acad. Dermatol.* 11:105–110, 1980.

5. Halprin K.M., Comerford M., Taylor J.R.: Constant low-dose ultraviolet light therapy for psoriasis. *J. Am. Acad. Dermatol.* 7:614–619, 1982.
6. Menkes A., Stern R.S., Arndt K.A.: Psoriasis treatment with suberythemogenic ultraviolet B radiation and a coal tar extract. *J. Am. Acad. Dermatol.* 12:21–25, 1984.
7. Adrian R.M., LeVine M.J., Parrish J.A.: Treatment frequency for outpatient phototherapy of psoriasis. A comparative study. *Arch. Dermatol.* 117:623–626, 1981.
8. LeVine M.J., Parrish J.A.: Outpatient phototherapy of psoriasis. *Arch. Dermatol.* 116:552–554, 1980.
9. Petrozzi J.W., Barton J.O., Kaidbey K.K., et al.: Updating the Goeckerman regimen for psoriasis. *Br. J. Dermatol.* 98:437–444, 1978.
10. Armstrong R.B., Leach E.E., Fleiss J.L., et al.: Modified Goeckerman therapy for psoriasis: A two-year follow-up of a combined hospital-ambulatory care program. *Arch. Dermatol.* 120:313–318, 1984.
11. Hebborn P., Cram D.: A new tar gel—dermatopharmacology and clinical efficacy, in Frost P., Gomez E.C. (eds.): *Recent Advances in Dermatopharmacology.* New York, Spectrum Publications, pp. 197–210, 1977.
12. Tannenbaum L., Parrish J.A., Pathak M.A.: Tar phototoxicity and phototherapy for psoriasis. *Arch. Dermatol.* 111:467–470, 1975.
13. LeVine M.J., White H.A.D., Parrish J.A.: Components of the Goeckerman regimen. *J. Invest. Dermatol.* 73:170–173, 1979.
14. Parrish J.A.: Phototherapy and photochemotherapy of skin diseases. *J. Invest. Dermatol.* 77:167–171, 1981.
15. Maibach H., Conant M.: Modified Goeckerman regimen: Decreased treatment time. *Arch. Dermatol.* 112:557, 1976.
16. Levine M.J., Parrish J.A.: The effect of topical fluocinonide ointment on phototherapy of psoriasis. *J. Invest. Dermatol.* 78:157–159, 1982.
17. Petrozzi J.W.: Topical steroids and UV radiation in psoriasis. *Arch. Dermatol.* 119:207–210, 1983.
18. Horwitz S., Johnson R., Sefton J., et al.: The addition of a topically applied corticosteroid to a modified Goeckerman regimen to treat psoriasis: The effect on duration of remission. Submitted for publication.
19. Larko O., Swanbeck G., Svartholm H.: The effect on psoriasis of clobetasol propionate used alone or in combination with UVB. *Acta Dermatol. Venereol.* 64:151–154, 1984.
20. Paul B.S., Momtaz-T. K., Stern R.S., et al.: Combined methotrexate-ultraviolet B therapy in the treatment of psoriasis. *J. Am. Acad. Dermatol.* 7:758–762, 1982.
21. Morison W.L., Momtaz-T. K., Parrish J.A., et al.: Combined methotrexate-PUVA therapy in the treatment of psoriasis. *J. Am. Acad. Dermatol.* 6:46–51, 1982.
22. Pittelkow M.R., Perry H.O., Muller S.A., et al.: Skin cancer in patients with psoriasis treated with coal tar. *Arch. Dermatol.* 117:465–468, 1981.
23. Menter A., Cram D.L.: The Goeckerman regimen in two psoriasis day care centers. *J. Am. Acad. Dermatol.* 9:59–65, 1983.
24. Stern R.S., Zierler S., Parrish J.A.: Skin carcinoma in patients with psoriasis treated with topical tar and artificial ultraviolet radiation. *Lancet* 1:732–735, 1980.
25. Stern R.S., Scotto J., Fears T.R.: Psoriasis and susceptibility to nonmelanoma skin cancer. *J. Am. Acad. Dermatol.* 12:67–73, 1985.

9 / Psoralen Phototherapy for Psoriasis

NICHOLAS J. LOWE, M.D., F.R.C.P., F.A.C.P.

THE PHOTOSENSITIZING drugs known as psoralens (P) and long wavelength (320–400 nm) ultraviolet light (UVA): (P + UVA = PUVA) have been successfully used in several countries for the treatment of psoriasis and certain other photoresponsive skin diseases (Plate 2).

Most of the studies in the United States have reported on the use of oral 8-methoxypsoralen and UVA. This is currently the form of PUVA most likely to be used in this country. Another form of PUVA delivery is a combination of topical 8-methoxypsoralen and UVA. This is sometimes a very practical and useful form of therapy for localized resistant psoriasis, particularly of the palms and soles.

In other countries other forms of psoralen phototherapy are used. These include oral 5-methoxypsoralen, used in Europe, and psoralen administered by bathing water, used in Scandinavia. Synthetic psoralens such as 5-methoxypsoralen are not available in this country, and this chapter will not refer to them further.

The purpose of this chapter, therefore, will be to define the practical aspects of 8-methoxypsoralen phototherapy for psoriasis.

PSORALEN PHOTOTHERAPY: BACKGROUND

Oral psoralens have been used for many years in the treatment of different skin diseases.[3] Psoralens obtained from plant sources have been used as a treatment for leukoderma and vitiligo for over two thousand years.[3] These drugs were first reported as being effective in the therapy of psoriasis in the early 1970s. One of the first reports of the use of PUVA using oral 8-methoxypsoralen in the treatment of psoriasis was published in 1974.[12] Subsequently, a long-term follow-up study has confirmed the efficacy of PUVA, but certain questions as regards long-term toxicity remain. The potential problems of long-term toxicity include an increased risk of skin carcinogenesis.[15]

The mechanisms of action of psoralen phototherapy in improving psoriasis are not clearly understood. It is known that some psoralens are able to intercalate with cellular DNA and to subsequently react with pyrimidine bases in a photocatalyzed reaction. It is possible that this may lead to a gradual suppression of the benign epidermal hyperplasia seen in psoriasis.

There are, however, several other potential mechanisms of action, including effects of PUVA on the inflammatory response present in psoriatic skin as well as a direct vascular effect. In addition, it is known that PUVA will influence certain immunologically mediated events, including the suppression of contact allergic dermatitis, and it leads to the reduction of identifiable Langerhans cells.

As noted previously, several different psoralen compounds have been used topically and orally for therapy of psoriasis. Some of the different psoralens are listed in Table 9–1.

The remainder of this chapter will deal principally with oral administration of 8-methoxypsoralen, as this remains probably the most frequently used form of therapy in the United States and Western Europe, although in France 5-methoxypsoralen is used extensively by the oral route and in Scandinavia bathwater delivery systems of 8-methoxypsoralen as well as trimethylpsoralen also are used with success.

ULTRAVIOLET SOURCES FOR USE WITH PSORALEN PHOTOTHERAPY

The reader is referred to Chapter 7, which reviews most of the important and available ultraviolet sources for phototherapy.

TABLE 9–1.—ORAL PSORALEN PHOTOTHERAPY:
FEATURES OF DIFFERENT PSORALENS

PSORALEN	FEATURES
8-methoxypsoralen (8 MOP)	Approved in U.S. and in Europe Erythemogenic Pruritis Nausea
5-methoxypsoralen (5 MOP)	Not approved in U.S. Available in Europe (France) Less erythemogenic ⎫ Less pruritus ⎬ than 8 MOP Less nausea ⎭
4-5-trimethylpsoralen	Available in U.S. and in Europe Poor response in psoriasis Effective for vitiligo repigmentation

Most available ultraviolet sources are broad-spectrum UVA fluorescent bulbs. These emit small amounts of UVB in addition to broad-range UVA, with most of the peak emission in UVA around 360–365 nm.

For practical purposes these are the only light sources appropriate for PUVA phototherapy currently available in most countries. The higher the intensity of UVA source, the shorter the treatment times required. Many different types of UVA units are available, among them upright cabinets containing 56 or more separate fluorescent tubes. Horizontal "lie-down" units are also available. Most patients are able to be treated in the vertical units, but the horizontal units are very useful for some elderly patients or patients who develop fainting episodes after long periods of standing.

Another practical problem which occurs with PUVA phototherapy units is that they produce significant heat and the patient can become very hot. It is therefore important that adequate ventilation be available and air conditioning be provided in the area of the phototherapy machine.

The output of the phototherapy fluorescent tubes gradually declines with usage and it is therefore most important that these are routinely monitored by an appropriate photodosimeter. In the author's phototherapy units we routinely monitor output every week and a flow sheet is attached to the front of the machine so that it is possible at a glance note the output of the tubes and modify the treatment times accordingly. We also regularly confirm spectral pattern using a spectral radiometer.

Some of the newer phototherapy machines have internal radiometer recorders that are attached to computerized devices. These continuously record the delivered UVA dosage and will stop the machine when the predetermined UVA dosage has been delivered. These are extremely valuable but in the author's experience should always be checked by a nurse technician who calculates the expected time for a UVA dose and checks the machine at that time to make sure that there has not been any malfunction of the computer control.

Finally, because of the thermal energy generated and the perspiration resulting in many patients, it is often practical to have an available shower for patients that may be used following their PUVA phototherapy.

PATIENT SELECTION FOR PUVA

Great care has to be taken to select patients for PUVA phototherapy because of the potential for long-term cumulative skin damage resulting from this form of therapy. Some of the indications for PUVA phototherapy in psoriasis are (1) severe or incapacitating psoriasis, (2) previous failure of conventional topical therapy, (3) previous failure of tar and ultraviolet phototherapy, and (4) rapid relapse after the above forms of therapy. Additionally, patients should be screened for conditions in which PUVA is contraindicated, such as (1) photosensitive diseases, (2) use of photosensitive drugs, (3) previous or present skin cancers, (4) previous x-ray therapy to the skin, or (5) cataracts. Additionally, women undergoing PUVA therapy should probably avoid pregnancy. Finally, ideally, patients receiving PUVA should not have skin type I.

In the author's opinion PUVA presently should be reserved for severe generalized psoriasis or psoriasis that is severe and incapacitating. This would include generalized pustular psoriasis, exfoliative psoriasis, and

TABLE 9–2.—Ophthalmology Examination Record for Patients Undergoing PUVA

To Ophthalmologist

For Patients Being Treated With Psoralen Phototherapy
OPHTHALMOLOGY EXAM RECORD

PATIENT: _____ DATE: _____

The above-mentioned patient is undergoing PUVA treatment (psoralen-ultraviolet A). An examination of the lens and retina is required of all PUVA patients. Your cooperation in recording your findings is greatly appreciated.

Please return to:

Nicholas J. Lowe, M.D., F.R.C.P., F.A.C.P.
Dermatology Program
University of California
Los Angeles, California 90024

1. Slit-lamp exam

2. Funduscopic exam

3. Visual acuity

4. Evidence of cataracts

_____ M.D.

Tel: _____

Address: _____

_____

_____

---

widespread plaque psoriasis that has failed to improve with other forms of therapy.

It is important to obtain certain data prior to starting a patient on PUVA. While it is not known that oral psoralens produce any problem of internal disease or hepatoxicity, it is still the author's habit of obtaining venous blood samples for a complete blood count, a full biochemistry panel (to include liver function tests), and ANA determination.

It should be noted that there is no evidence at present that PUVA induces lupus erythematosus or a significant increase in antinuclear antibodies. It is clearly unwise for lupus patients to receive phototherapy. It should be noted that lupus erythematosus can mimic psoriasis in some patients.

Patients should receive a complete ophthalmologic examination and the ophthalmologist should be particularly aware of the concern for ocular disease (Table 9–2).

All patients taking oral psoralens need to be carefully instructed about the use of protective eyeglasses, which should be worn for the remainder of the day of treatment when the patient is out of doors or exposed to sunlight near window glass. It is particularly important to stress to patients that even when they are sitting by an unshielded window or driving a car for the remainder of the day of treatment they must wear their protective glasses. In addition, a list of some suitable protective eyeglasses should be given to the patient. Ultraviolet absorption of any glasses can be checked using a photodosimeter and the UVA machine. The glasses, if they are to be safely used, should block UVA transmission.

All patients undergoing PUVA should receive thorough instructions about the therapy, about potential side effects, and about precautions against side effects. The following sample instructions are used in our practice.

USEFUL INFORMATION FOR THE PATIENT PRIOR TO ORAL PUVA PHOTOCHEMOTHERAPY

Photochemotherapy is a treatment program for various cutaneous problems including psoriasis, lichen planus, vitiligo, various eczematous conditions and mycosis fungoides. This therapy involves a combination of psoralens and a special form of ultraviolet light provided by light from a high-energy source. This program has been nicknamed *PUVA* therapy, *P* standing for psoralen and the *UVA* for the spectrum of ultraviolet light provided by special lights. This approach has been used by a large number of centers throughout Europe and several centers in the United States. The treatment is not a cure—it is a control. The purpose of the treatment is to create a clearing of the condition sufficient for the patient to maintain the skin in a controlled, relatively clear state with topical preparations used at home. The program involves taking oral psoralen capsules according to your weight two hours before your treatment time. The special light treatment is not effective without the psoralen capsules, which create a photosensitivity of the skin, enabling the light to affect the dermatitis.

NOTE: Pregnant women should not be treated. The psoralen capsules have not been proven safe for use during pregnancy. In addition, women are advised to be using conventional methods of birth control while taking part in this PUVA program.

An eye examination by an ophthalmologist (eye specialist) will be arranged prior to the beginning of the program and again at six to eight months after the treatment is started. This is done to insure that there are no eye conditions that would preclude the patient taking part in the photo treatment program, even though we would be using special plastic gray or green sunglasses on the day of the treatment program and during the light therapy.

Possible Side-Effects With Oral Psoralens

1. Occasional nausea and stomach upset (in about 10% of patients). This can often be corrected by taking pills with food or milk.

2. An exaggerated sunburn. The medication stays in the skin for approximately eight hours after it has been taken; therefore, it is important to avoid sun exposure after the treatment by the use of physical protection with clothing and chemical sunscreens.

The treatment may cause a sunburn-type of reaction but this is usually prevented by controlling the dosage of psoralens and the length of time in the light box.

3. Pigmentation of the skin. Patients will have a moderate to deep suntan, which usually fades within six to eight weeks after cessation of the therapy.

4. The eyes will be more sensitive to the light during the treatment. For eight hours after you have taken the medication, you should wear green or gray plastic protective sunglasses if you are outside. Although no long-term side effects to the eyes are known, this type of precaution seems sensible.

5. Unforeseen effects: Although all the known possible side effects have been reviewed, there may be complications or reactions that could arise

from this therapy. This situation exists with all new treatment programs and must be recognized and accepted by the participants. It is possible with any form of ultraviolet treatment that an increased incidence of skin cancer may be seen later in some patients. This may particularly occur in patients who are fair-skinned or have had previous radiation therapy for their skin disease.

Each patient will vary in the number of treatments per week and the number of weeks it will take to reach clearing. It is estimated that the average patient will require two or three treatments each week. Initially the treatment will start with only a few minutes of light and then gradually be increased to a tolerance level. Clearing takes an average of 15 to 20 treatments. After clearing some patients may be maintained at a relatively clear state with one treatment every one to four weeks. There is a great deal of individual variation and there is no way I can tell what your schedule will be until you are well into the treatment program.

Although PUVA was approved in the United States for therapy of psoriasis in 1982, the author still feels it is wise to have patients read, hopefully understand, and sign an appropriate informed consent form. This may help to insure that they understand the potential risks of this therapy. An example of such an informed consent form is given in Table 9–3.

DETERMINATION OF INITIAL PUVA DOSAGE

Having selected the appropriate patient for PUVA therapy the guidelines for determining initial patient dosage are as follows.

Drug Doses

The dosage of oral 8-methoxypsoralen is usually calculated on a dose of 0.6 mg per kg body weight, taken as 10 mg capsules (Table 9–4). There are for practical purposes two alternative forms of oral 8-methoxypsoralen currently available in the United States. There are likely to be several other forms available in Europe. In the United States the existing methoxsalen (Elder) is apparently absorbed at a slower rate than some of the newer forms of oral 8-methoxypsoralen, such as the HOUVA methoxsalen capsules (National Biological).

The author has recently been involved in a comparative study of a more rapidly absorbable form of methoxsalen in capsules as compared to the older form. Both forms of methoxsalen were supplied by Elder Pharma-

TABLE 9–3.—Oral Psoralen Photochemotherapy Patient Consent Form

I understand that I will be treated with a drug called psoralen. This treatment consists of taking psoralen capsules orally two hours prior to exposure to a high-intensity long-wave ultraviolet lamp system. The purpose of this study is to evaluate further this form of treatment in my skin disease.

I understand that psoralen, in combination with long-wave ultraviolet light, recently has been approved by the U.S. Food and Drug Administration (FDA) as an effective treatment for psoriasis. It is my understanding that the side effects and potential toxicity associated with this treatment have been explained to me and may be listed as follows: Early side effects occasionally include increased itching and redness of the skin, which may occasionally develop into excessive redness or burning. A very small percentage of patients develop nausea after ingesting the tablets. Very occasionally, the use of a tablet to control nausea may be necessary. Potential long-term risks of PUVA, such as premature skin aging, development of cataracts, and induction of skin malignancies, remain a possibility. As with all treatment, some patients may fail to improve despite treatment. The potential benefit of this form of treatment is that my skin disease will be significantly improved.

In addition, I understand that a complete eye examination will be done prior to therapy and at regular intervals while continuing psoralen photochemotherapy. The purpose of this eye examination is to exclude the possibility of cataracts or other eye abnormalities. I have been advised to wear protective eyeglasses before, during and after PUVA on the day of treatment only. In addition, I understand that I also should avoid sun exposure on the day of treatment.

I further understand that I should not participate in this program if I am pregnant or might be and should I become pregnant I should inform the doctor conducting the study immediately and stop using the medication. I understand it is vital that female subjects do not try to become pregnant while undergoing this treatment.

I understand a small skin biopsy may be taken from normally covered skin prior to treatment and that this may be repeated to assess any effects of treatment. This skin biopsy will not benefit me directly but will assist in evaluation of the treatment. I also understand that before treatment, 45 cc of blood (approx. 4 teaspoonfuls) will be drawn. This may be repeated about every 6–12 months of treatment.

I understand I may contact my doctor at the telephone number provided if I have any questions regarding my treatment.

I understand this treatment will be continued until the skin disease has improved significantly or cleared. Then I either will be placed on less frequent treatments to control the skin disease or the treatment will be stopped. I understand each patient is expected to respond at a different individual rate to treatments.

Signature of Patient   Date

Physician

---

ceuticals, Bryan, Ohio. The lesions of patients treated with the more rapidly absorbed form of 8-methoxypsoralen cleared at a significantly faster pace than those of patients using the older form of the drug, and more patients achieved improvement with the more rapidly absorbable drug.

It is to be hoped that further refinements of these different forms of 8-methoxypsoralen will insure standardization and optimized therapeutic responses. It has been noted that peak serum 8-methoxypsoralen levels may vary greatly between patients and that the time for the psoralen peak to be

TABLE 9–4.—Guidelines
for Determining Psoralen
Oral Doses

| PATIENT WEIGHT | | PSORALEN DOSE |
kg	lb	(mg)
< 30	< 65	10
30–50	66–110	20
51–65	111–145	30
66–80	146–175	40
81–90	176–200	50
91–115	201–250	60
> 115	> 250	70

achieved may vary from 1–6 hours.[5] Some newer forms of 8-methoxypso-
ralen are liquid formulations, compared to the older forms, which are crys-
talline formulations.

Selection of Initial UVA Dosage

There are two ways of determining the initial UVA dosage. The simplest
and most rapid way is to use a history of the patient's skin type responses
to sunlight exposure. These responses, together with the suggested initial
UVA dose, are given in Table 9–5.

An alternative way of determining the initial dosage is to obtain the minimal phototoxic dose (MPD) required to produce visual erythema. The patient takes the oral dose of psoralen and two hours after this is placed in
the UVA machine and has areas of skin exposed to incremental amounts of
UVA. In the author's experience the MPD is a safe way of determining the

TABLE 9–5.—Skin Types and Responses
to Previous Sun Exposures Used to
Determine Initial UVA Exposures

SKIN TYPE	ESTIMATED INITIAL UVA DOSE* (J/sq cm)
I. Always Burn, Never Tan	1.0
II. Always Burn, Sometimes Tan	2.0
III. Sometimes Burn, Always Tan	3.0
IV. Never Burns, Tans Readily	4.0
V. Moderate Pigmentation	5.0
VI. Marked Pigmentation	6.0

*UVA usually given 2 hours after oral 8-methoxypso-
ralen, 0.6 mg/kg.

safe initial UVA dosage, particularly in patients who may have a lighter skin type and a history of previous sunburn or photosensitive skin reactions. The author usually has these patients tested at 1, 3, 5, 7, and 9 J/sq cm by using templates applied to the skin and the exposure of 1 sq cm areas of skin.

The skin should be examined at 48 and ideally at 72 hours to determine minimum phototoxic response prior to embarking on the selection of initial UVA dosing of whole body therapy.

SUBSEQUENT PUVA THERAPY

The initial psoralen and UVA dose having been determined, the patient then usually is treated as frequently as possible to obtain a maximum response. In practical terms, this should be no more frequent in most patients than Mondays, Wednesdays, and Fridays. The reason for this is that it takes at least 48 hours and in some patients longer to develop a maximum phototoxic erythema. It is therefore safer to treat no more frequently than every other day. Some patients because of problems of transportation and distance may not be able to receive treatments as frequently as this. It is important to advise these patients that their improvement may take longer than if they were able to be treated on a more frequent basis.

It is usual to increase the amount of UVA at each treatment unless there is any evidence of skin side effects such as pruritus or phototoxic erythema. The usual dose increase is between 0.5 and 2 J/sq cm, dependent on the absence of skin side effects, the response of the psoriasis, and the skin type. Recent reports have suggested that more frequent PUVA is possible in some patients and it is the author's impression that darker skin types can tolerate two consecutive days of PUVA followed by a rest day.

In addition, PUVA has been combined with UVB phototherapy, giving an apparently enhanced clearing rate in selected patients.[11] Again, in the author's experience this is particularly useful for patients with darker skin types or with chronic recalcitrant plaque psoriasis. It is more hazardous in patients with lighter skin types and more severe or unstable forms of psoriasis.

Adjunctive Therapy With PUVA

It is possible to combine PUVA therapy with other forms of antipsoriatic therapy and obtain an enhanced response. These forms of adjunctive therapy have included such topical agents as cortiosteroids[10] and anthralin.[2] In addition, combination therapy with systemic antipsoriatic agents and PUVA also has been described. There has apparently been good success in combining oral aromatic retinoids (Etretinate in the United States and Tigason in Europe) with PUVA.[4, 7]

Whether or not other forms of synthetic retinoids may be combined with PUVA remains to be determined. In the author's experience 13-cis-retinoic acid, which is an extremely effective synthetic retinoid for treatment of severe forms of acne, has a disappointing effect on the treatment of psoriasis. There are, however, some patients who develop resistance or do not clear completely with PUVA, who show an enhanced response with the addition of 13-cis-retinoic acid and continued PUVA. Unfortunately, however, this only occurs in a small percentage of patients.

MAINTENANCE PUVA PHOTOTHERAPY

Maintenance PUVA therapy should be performed at the minimum rate to control the patient's disease. In view of the evidence for cumulative PUVA skin toxicity,[14] it is important to constantly extend the time periods between PUVA treatments. In addition, it is important where possible to discontinue PUVA therapy once the maximum response has been achieved. Some patients do have reasonable remission times after stopping PUVA[2] but many require some form of maintenance therapy.

Careful, regular follow-up examination by the dermatologist is necessary when the patient is on a maintenance PUVA program. In particular, when higher amounts of UVA have been delivered (1,000 J/sq cm and above), careful scrutiny for presence of early skin cancers is necessary.

Repeat ophthalmic and hematologic examinations probably should be performed approximately every year if the patient is on a regular maintenance program.

ALTERNATIVE FORMS OF PUVA THERAPY

Psoralens other than 8-methoxypsoralen have been suggested as being effective alternatives in PUVA phototherapy. In particular, 5-methoxypsoralen has been studied extensively in France and has been suggested to be less erythemogenic and to produce less nausea and pruritus than 8-methoxypsoralen. No controlled studies have been performed in this country, however.

Topical Psoralen Delivery

Another form of psoralen, 3-carbethoxypsoralen, has been suggested as being effective, noncarcinogenic and producing no phototoxic erythema. Again, these reports have as yet to be confirmed.

Topical psoralens have been studied and have been shown to be useful in the treatment of localized forms of the disease when applied usually in an ointment form.[13] However, in the author's experience the problems that may result from this form of topical psoralen therapy are an uneven response, patchy hyperpigmentation and an increased risk of unwanted phototoxic erythema and blistering.

An alternative way of delivering psoralens has been examined in Scandinavia, where both 8-methoxypsoralen and trimethyl-psoralen have been delivered in bathwater. A very dilute psoralen solution is made in the bathwater; the patient soaks in the psoralen bath for 15 minutes, then undergoes UVA phototherapy.

Potential advantages for topical psoralens are that higher skin levels of the drug are achievable, thereby requiring much lower amounts of UVA to produce the required therapeutic response. In the author's experience, often one tenth of the UVA required for oral PUVA is necessary for topical PUVA. In an unpublished study of minimal phototoxic doses from 0.1% 8-methoxypsoralen in an alcoholic vehicle, the MPD ranged from 0.3–0.7 J/sq cm. This is approximately one tenth of the MPD range seen after oral 8-methoxypsoralen; therefore, much faster and shorter treatments are possible.

The potential disadvantages are the persistence of the psoralens in the skin, leading to the risk of persistent and severe phototoxicity. This can occur, for example, two or three days after the topical psoralen treatment, should the patient's skin be exposed to the sun. The author has seen numerous examples where patients have developed phototoxic blisters following sun exposures several days after topical psoralen application. In addition, the long-term risk of cutaneous malignancy with topical psoralens may be different from oral psoralens. On the other hand, with smaller amounts of UVA being delivered to the skin during topical psoralen therapy it is possible that we may see less chronic actinic damage. These questions need to be reexamined and, it is hoped, answered in the future.

Table 9–6 summarizes the advantages and disadvantages of topical psoralen therapy.

TABLE 9–6.—ADVANTAGES AND DISADVANTAGES OF TOPICALLY
ADMINISTERED PSORALENS

TYPE OF PREPARATION	ADVANTAGES	DISADVANTAGES
Psoralen lotions, creams, or ointments*	No systemic side effects Rapid UVA-induced phototherapeutic effects with short treatment times Probably no ocular effects	Easy phototoxicity Persistance in skin Not uniformly applied: variable response and pigmentation Unknown relative skin carcinogenic risk
Psoralens by bathwater delivery	Uniform skin delivery Short UVA radiation times No systemic side effects Probably no ocular effects	Unknown relative skin carcinogenic risk Specialized bathing facilities are needed

*In U.S., 8-methoxypsoralen, usual concentration 0.1%–1.0%, in hydroalcoholic lotions, creams, or ointments.

SIDE EFFECTS OF PUVA PHOTOTHERAPY (TABLE 9–7)

Early Side Effects

The early side effects of PUVA phototherapy include the undesired effects of phototoxic erythema, increased pruritus, the occurrence of nausea and the appearance of variable pigmentation, particularly hyper- and hypopigmentation. Hyperpigmentation in particular can be a problem in women who have previous chloasma. The use of broad spectrum sunscreens and shielding of uninvolved skin may help to reduce some skin side effects. We, for example, frequently cover the face with broad-range sunscreens as well as light-proof toweling if there is no psoriasis affecting the face.

In addition to these side effects, some patients' psoriasis will get worse with any form of phototherapy, including PUVA.

Occasionally patients will also complain of other vague symptoms, in-

TABLE 9–7.—POSSIBLE SIDE EFFECTS
OF PUVA

EARLY	LATE
Phototoxic erythema	Skin carcinogenesis
Pruritus	Enhanced skin aging
Nausea	Pigmentary changes
Worsening of psoriasis	Ocular damage

cluding light-headedness, headache, disorientation, and diarrhea. It is often difficult to determine clearly whether the PUVA has caused these side effects.

Patients may be anxious about being in an enclosed cabinet for significant lengths of time, particularly patients who have a degree of claustrophobia.

All of these potential concerns should be fully discussed with the patient should they occur. Some of the newer UVA machines are less enclosed— for example, the Psoralite machine—and thus may be more acceptable for the patient who does not wish to be so confined for the treatment time.

Delayed Side Effects

The delayed side effects of PUVA are of major concern and are the reason why the treatment should be reserved for older patients with severe skin disease. It is known, for example, that PUVA can induce short-term and long-term changes in immune responses. These include decreased viability of lymphocytes and suppressed reactivity in in vitro lymphocyte testing. We are unclear of the long-term implications of these immunologic changes. It is possible that they may be partly involved in increasing the risk of skin tumors seen in patients treated with PUVA.

Nonmelanoma Skin Cancer From PUVA

It has been shown that PUVA is photomutagenic in different bacterial strains. In addition, it has been shown in several animal studies that psoralens and UVA are capable of inducing multiple skin cancers in mice.[1]

Recent studies have confirmed that there is an increased relative risk of squamous cell carcinoma arising in patients treated with chronic PUVA.[6, 15] There was apparently less increase in basal cell carcinoma in this group. Other studies have failed to show an increase in skin cancers.[14]

Caution needs to be exercised concerning patients to whom long-term cumulative PUVA radiation has been delivered. These patients, if they have the lighter skin types I and II, may be at significant risk for skin cancers. It is important even if PUVA therapy has been discontinued for patients who have received significant amounts of PUVA to have regular follow-up examinations to exclude the possibility of skin cancer formation.

Melanocyte Effects

Psoralens are known to stimulate melanogenesis. Recent studies have reported the occurrence of melanoma and also dysplastic melanocytes in patients treated with PUVA, however at this stage there have been no reports from the multicenter studies of an increased incidence of melanoma.[15] Clearly patients need to be followed carefully and examined for the possibility of induction of malignant melanoma.

PUVA and Skin Aging

Repeated phototoxic injury to the skin can produce dermal changes that may be important as mechanisms of skin and dermal aging. Recent studies in the mouse have suggested that repeated UVA exposures alter dermal collagen and elastin metabolism. In addition, persistent elastic tissue changes have been observed in the skin following PUVA phototherapy.[16]

The long-term extent and significance of these alterations remain to be determined.

Ocular Damage

While there are theoretical reasons to suspect human lens photodegeneration leading to cataract formation,[7] (which has been reported in rabbits), there does not seem to be an increased risk of cataract formation in patients treated with PUVA.[14, 15] One possible reason for this is the careful use of photoprotective eyeglasses.

SUMMARY OF PUVA THERAPY

PUVA phototherapy represents an effective and valuable form of therapy in carefully selected patients who have more severe forms of psoriasis. It is not a treatment that should be used without consideration of all possible factors itemized in this chapter.

For the patient, it has many advantages over messy topical forms of therapy. It should not, however, be used as a substitute for topical therapy unless there are clear indications.

The patient should be fully informed at all times of the potential hazards with PUVA and in the author's experience should always be given full information on this form of therapy. Newer refinements of psoralen phototherapy could include improvement in topical delivery of the drugs and possible "targeting" of the psoralens to the epidermis after oral therapy.

REFERENCES

1. Griffin A.R., Hakim R.E., Knox J.M.: Erythema and tumor formulation in methoxsalen treated mice exposed to fluorescent light. *Arch. Dermatol.* 82:572–577, 1966.
2. Cripps D.J., Lowe N.J.: Photochemotherapy for psoriasis remission times. Psoralen and UVA and combined photochemotherapy with anthralin. *Clin. Exp. Dermatol.* 4:477–483, 1979.
3. Fitzpatrick T.B., Pathak M.A.: Historical aspects of methoxsalen and furocoumarins. *J. Invest. Dermatol.* 32:225–228, 1959.
4. Fritsch P.O., Honigsmann H., Jaschke E., et al.: Augmentation of oral methoxsalen-photochemotherapy with an oral retinoic acid derivative. *J. Invest. Dermatol.* 70:178–182, 1978.
5. Goldstein D.P., Carter D.M., Ljuggren B., et al.: Minimal phototoxic doses and 8-MOP plasma levels in PUVA patients. *J. Invest. Dermatol.* 78:429–433, 1982.
6. Honigsmann H., Wolff K., Gschnait F., et al.: Keratosis and nonmelanoma skin tumors in long-term photochemotherapy (PUVA). *J. Am. Acad. Dermatol.* 3:406–414, 1980.
7. Lauharanta J., Juvakoski T., Lassus A.: A clinical evaluation of the effects of an aromatic retinoid (Tigason) combination of retinoid and PUVA, and PUVA alone in severe psoriasis. *Br. J. Dermatol.* 104:325, 1981.
8. Lerman S., Megaw J., Willis I.: Potential ocular complications for PUVA therapy and their prevention. *J. Inst. Dermatol.* 74:197–199, 1980.
9. Melski J.W., Tannenbaum L., Parrish J.A., et al.: Oral methoxsalen photochemotherapy for the treatment of psoriasis: A cooperative clinical trial. *J. Invest. Dermatol.* 68:328–335, 1977.
10. Morison W.L., Parrish J.A., Fitzpatrick T.B.: Controlled study of PUVA and adjunctive topical therapy in the management of psoriasis. *Br. J. Dermatol.* 98:125–132, 1978.
11. Parrish J.A.: Phototherapy and photochemotherapy of skin diseases. *J. Invest. Dermatol.* 77:1657–171, 1981.
12. Parrish J.A., Fitzpatrick T.B., Tannenbaum L., et al.: Photochemotherapy of psoriasis with oral methoxsalen and long wavelength ultraviolet light. *N. Engl. J. Med.* 291:1207–1212, 1974.
13. Petrozzi J.W., Kaidbey K.M., Kligman A.M.: Topical methoxsalen and blacklight in the treatment of psoriasis. *Arch. Dermatol.* 113:292–296, 1977.
14. Roenigk H.H., Farber E.M., Storrs F., et al.: Photochemotherapy for psoriasis: A clinical cooperative study of PUVA-48 and PUVA-64. *Arch. Dermatol.* 115:576–579, 1979.
15. Stern R.S., Thibodeau L.A., Kleinerman R.A., et al.: Risk factors and increased incidence of cutaneous carcinoma in patients treated with oral methoxsalen photochemotherapy for psoriasis. *N. Engl. J. Med.* 300:809–813, 1979.
16. Zelickson A.S., Mottaz J.H., Zelickson B.D., et al.: Elastic tissue changes in skin following PUVA therapy. *J. Am. Acad. Dermatol.* 3:186–192, 1980.

10 / Systemic Chemotherapy for Psoriasis

MARY E. HARTMAN, M.D.
GERALD D. WEINSTEIN, M.D.

PSORIASIS IS generally considered a benign disease whose major importance to the patient is cosmetic and psychologic. Systemic chemotherapy or any potentially toxic therapy, therefore, should be reserved for severe psoriasis. Simpler and potentially less toxic therapies should be tried first, including phototherapy with tars and UVB, as well as PUVA. When the psoriasis is unresponsive to these therapies and is life-threatening or incapacitating physically, emotionally, or economically, agents such as methotrexate, when properly used, can produce excellent clinical benefit with very few side effects.

Systemic chemotherapy is not a cure for psoriasis, but it is a valuable therapeutic approach to control the signs and symptoms of the disease. The goal of treatment should be maximal improvement with the lowest dose possible, rather than using higher doses to achieve total clinical clearing. Also, extended rest periods from systemic therapy should be used whenever possible. For example, in a given patient systemic chemotherapy may be interrupted during the summertime when the patient could be encouraged to use sunlight to help control his psoriasis.

The first systemic chemotherapeutic agent administered for psoriasis was the folic acid antagonist aminopterin. It was first used for the therapy of leukemia and found serendipitiously to be effective in psoriasis. Methotrexate, a close analogue of aminopterin, replaced aminopterin to become the only systemic drug approved in the United States for the treatment of psoriasis, and thus is the standard of comparison for any new systemic agent.

99

PATHOPHYSIOLOGIC BASIS FOR CHEMOTHERAPY IN PSORIASIS

Psoriasis is characterized by excessive and rapid proliferation of epidermal cells. Cell kinetic studies now show that psoriatic epidermal cells have a cell cycle of 36 hours; the cycle in normal epidermis is eight times longer. The number of proliferative cells in psoriasis is double the number in normal epidermis. The combination of these factors yields a production of 25,000 cells per square millimeter of surface area per day in psoriasis, compared to only 1,400 cells in normal skin. Also, psoriatic skin contains eight times the number of cells in S (synthesis) phase of cell division at any time.[27] This is an ideal target for therapeutic modalities that interfere with cell proliferation.

METHOTREXATE MECHANISM OF ACTION

Methotrexate acts on proliferating cells by inhibiting the S phase. The folic acid antagonists inhibit dihydrofolic reductase, an enzyme required to provide methyl donor groups for the synthesis of DNA, RNA, and protein. The pathway most affected by methotrexate is the synthesis of thymidylate, one of the four precursors of DNA. Without adequate thymidylate, DNA synthesis is inhibited and cell division is halted in the affected cells. Besides blocking the abnormal rapid proliferation of psoriasis, methotrexate affects other normally rapidly growing tissues such as bone marrow, gastrointestinal tissues and hair roots.

In psoriasis, methotrexate appears to be acting directly on the epidermal cells rather than on a distant target. Following systemic or intralesional administration of methotrexate, DNA synthesis and mitotic activity abruptly stop in epidermal cells.[25] Psoriatic skin is more sensitive than normal skin to methotrexate's activity for at least two reasons: the fact that eight-fold more psoriatic cells than normal cells are in S phase and the fact that psoriatic cells have an increased dependence on the de novo thymidylate pathway while normal epidermal cells can bypass this block with the salvage pathway.[9]

CLINICAL ASPECTS

Methotrexate was prescribed for patients with psoriasis by 52% of 510 dermatologists surveyed in 1974.[3] The widespread availability of PUVA has

TABLE 10–1.—Indications for
Systemic Therapy for Psoriasis

Psoriatic erythroderma
Acute pustular psoriasis
Localized pustular psoriasis
Psoriatic arthritis
Extensive psoriasis unresponsive to other, less
    toxic therapies
Psoriasis in areas preventing the individual from
    obtaining gainful employment
Psoriasis that is severely disabling psychologically

undoubtedly reduced the number of patients receiving methotrexate, but it continues to be a valuable therapeutic tool for patients with severe psoriasis.

The selection of patients for methotrexate therapy is based on indications relative to the severity of the psoriasis (Table 10–1) and considering the relative contraindications of the drug (Table 10–2). Within these guidelines, the therapy of each patient must be individualized to carefully weigh benefits versus risks.

The clinical benefits of methotrexate for psoriatic arthritis were recently confirmed in a double-blind study.[7] Methotrexate remains the drug of choice for severe and otherwise unresponsive seronegative psoriatic arthritis, even with minimal skin involvement.

Prior to initiating therapy, emphasis is placed on evaluating renal and liver functions. Methotrexate is excreted mainly via the kidneys, which is of particular concern in older individuals who tend to have reduced creatinine clearances and therefore clinically require lower doses of methotrexate than do younger patients. Liver function is evaluated in four ways to determine the presence of preexisting disease:

TABLE 2.—Relative Contraindications for Methotrexate Therapy

Significantly decreased renal function
Significantly abnormal liver function
Pregnancy (absolute)
Patient (male or female) planning on conceiving a child: conception should be avoided for at
    least 12 weeks after methotrexate has been stopped
Recent or active hepatitis
Cirrhosis
Excessive alcohol consumption
Severe leukopenia, thrombocytopenia, or anemia
Active peptic ulcer (near absolute)
Active, severe infectious diseases
Unreliable patient

These contraindications may be waived in a given patient if the benefits of therapy will outweigh the risks that may be incurred.

1. A careful history is obtained to rule out risk factors for liver disease, such as excessive alcohol consumption, exposure to arsenic, previous hepatitis or jaundice, diabetes mellitus, chronic congestive heart failure, and ileojejunal bypass surgery for obesity.

2. A physical examination is performed, including examining the liver as well as cutaneous findings associated with cirrhosis.

3. The standard liver function tests are obtained, including SGOT, SGPT, and alkaline phosphatase. Unfortunately, these are not completely reliable in detecting severe liver disease. In a high percentage of biopsy-proven fibrosis or cirrhosis cases, the laboratory tests have been within normal limits.[26]

4. It is necessary to perform a liver biopsy in the majority of patients prior to starting methotrexate. Radioisotope liver scans are not recommended for routinely evaluating the liver because they have failed to be as accurate as the liver biopsy.[4]

Table 10–3 summarizes the procedures necessary for monitoring patients undergoing methotrexate therapy. Suggested instructions for patients are shown in Table 10–4.

DOSAGE

Schedules for methotrexate delivery were derived empirically, starting with the small daily dosage schedule[15] and followed by the weekly

TABLE 10–3.—MONITORING NECESSARY FOR METHOTREXATE THERAPY

Pretherapy evaluation
  History and physical examination
  Complete blood cell count with platelet count
  Renal function tests
    Urinalysis
    BUN
    24-hour urine for creatinine clearance
    Serum creatinine
  Liver function tests
    SGOT
    SGPT
    Alkaline phosphatase
  Chest x-ray
  Liver biopsy
Ongoing therapy
  Leukocyte and platelet count (every 1–4 weeks at least one week after the last dose)
  Hemoglobin, urinalysis, serum creatinine, liver function tests (every 3–4 months, at least one week after the last dose)
  Chest x-ray (yearly)
  Liver biopsy (after every 1.5 gm cumulative methotrexate dose, at least two weeks after the last dose, with more frequent liver biopsies—every 1.0 gm cumulative dose—if there are one or more cirrhosis risk factors present, significant liver function abnormalities, or signs of liver disease are present)

Table 10–4.—Instructions for Patients Undergoing Methotrexate Therapy

Very often effective for *severe or resistant psoriasis*
Often effective for *psoriatic arthritis*
How is it taken?
  Usually once-weekly oral doses; it may be given by injection to some patients
Great care is needed when taking methotrexate
Before treatment
  Careful history and examination by physician
  Blood and urine tests
  Liver biopsy (usually overnight hospitalization)
During treatment
  Take *correct dose* of drug at the *same time and day* each week
  Do *not* increase dose yourself
  Avoid alcohol
  Avoid other drugs (ask physician prior to taking any other medication)
  If you have *any problems* with *sore throat, skin or any infections, skin ulcers or mouth ulcers*
  STOP METHOTREXATE AND CALL PHYSICIAN
  See physician regularly, usually every 4 weeks
  Physician visits and blood tests will be required more often in early stages of methotrexate therapy.

intramuscular[21] or oral dose schedules.[16] In 1971 the triple-dose regimen was proposed, based on the psoriatic cell cycle.[24] On this schedule the patient takes three doses orally at 12-hour intervals each week. Since therapeutic methotrexate blood levels as well as DNA synthesis inhibition in psoriatic cells are present for 6–14 hours after each dose administered,[5, 25] there is a putative therapeutic effect for the entire 36-hour psoriatic cell cycle. The triple-dose schedule has less real and theoretic toxicity but equal effectivenss of the other schedules.

On the triple-dose schedule patients are started (after a test dose of 5 mg) on one 2.5 mg tablet orally at 12-hour intervals for three doses only. The next week the dosage is increased by one tablet so that the patient takes two tablets (hour 0), one tablet (hour 12) and one tablet (hour 24), for a total dose of 10 mg. In subsequent weeks the dose is titrated up or down by a 2.5 mg tablet to the most effective and best-tolerated dose. This is usually achieved by the two-tablet, two-tablet, two-tablet dosage for a total of 15 mg/week. This dosage is maintained until the desired degree of clearing is obtained. Infrequently a higher dose is required for larger patients or more resistant psoriasis.

The single weekly oral dose schedule starts with a 5–7.5 mg test dose and then is increased by 2.5 mg increments per week. The dosage range is generally between 7.5 and 25 mg per week, with rare patients requiring up to 37.5 mg per week. Intramuscular dose schedules are infrequently used, usually for unreliable patients. Intramuscular doses are given weekly and are somewhat higher than the oral doses because blood levels are not sustained as long as after oral doses.

MONITORING THERAPY

During therapy, leukocyte and platelet counts are maximally depressed about one week following drug administration. A drop in these counts below minimal normal levels generally necessitates reducing dosage or temporarily discontinuing therapy. Early clinical experience with methotrexate (or aminopterin) used the presence of oral ulcerations in a patient to indicate too high a dosage of drug. Today, oral ulcerations are rarely seen as a side effect of methotrexate in the treatment of psoriasis due to lower doses and careful monitoring of blood counts every one to four weeks.

Liver function tests are obtained at 3–4 month intervals, but at least one week after the last dose of the drug. Methotrexate causes transient elevations in liver function tests for 1–3 days after its administration. If significant liver function abnormalities are present at one week after the last dose, methotrexate should be discontinued for 1 to 2 weeks and the tests repeated. Persistent abnormalities warrant a liver biopsy in most cases.

SIDE EFFECTS

Methotrexate is recommended for only a select group of severely psoriatic patients because of warranted concern about potential severe liver toxicity. Six studies examining liver biopsies of a total of 309 patients before and after methotrexate treatment showed approximately 3% developed cirrhosis.[26] Cumulative doses of 4 gm or more have led to an incidence as high as 25% (Table 10–5). The incidence of methotrexate-induced cirrhosis in the United States appears to be lower than in the Scandinavian popula-

TABLE 10–5.—INCIDENCE OF METHOTREXATE-RELATED CIRRHOSIS IN PATIENTS WITH PRE- AND POSTTREATMENT LIVER BIOPSIES

AUTHOR	YEAR	NUMBER OF PATIENTS	CUMULATIVE DOSE (mg)	PATIENTS WITH CIRRHOSIS (%)
Weinstein[26]	1973	81	2232	0
Zachariae[28]	1975	96	1164	6
Warin[23]	1975	25	750	0
Nyfors[13]	1976	88	1733	6
Zachariae[30]	1980	96	2200	13.5
Zachariae[30]	1980	39	>4000	25.6
Ashton[1]	1982	36	1955	5

tions reported by Zachariae (H. Zachariae, personal communication) and Nyfors.[13]

There are several major considerations regarding liver toxicity with methotrexate therapy. Severe liver disease, such as fibrosis and cirrhosis, could be present in patients with psoriasis, at the same incidence as in the general public, before the administration of methotrexate. Heavy intake of alcohol is a significant factor in the development of severe liver toxicity. No liver function tests are reliable indicators of liver disease. In patients with a cumulative methotrexate dose less than 1.5 gm the risk of cirrhosis is relatively low, but the risk may increase when higher cumulative doses, in the range of 4.0 gm, are reached.

Other risk factors for development of cirrhosis on methotrexate include obesity, diabetes, lowered renal function, and preexisting liver pathology. The risk of severe liver toxicity may be reduced by titrating the patient to the lowest possible dose to achieve and maintain adequate control, rather than 100% clearing, of the psoriasis. When the patient is doing well on a maintenance regime, intervals between doses may be increased from 7 days to 10–14 days, with several-month rest periods when possible. These guidelines can permit a longer-term use of methotrexate. Also, the patient should be warned to avoid ethanol consumption if possible.

Recommendations for future methotrexate treatment are made on the basis of the histologic changes found in the liver. It is therefore advisable to make your local pathologist aware of the methotrexate guidelines reference.[16] The classification of the pathologic changes of the liver are listed in Table 10–6. If moderate to severe fibrosis or cirrhosis appears on liver biopsy, then treatment with methotrexate should be curtailed. In a study by Zachariae, however, patients who had documented cirrhosis were continued on methotrexate with most cases showing little to no worsening in liver pathology by biopsy and a few patients actually showing improvement.[30] This indicates methotrexate cirrhosis may be a less aggressive disease than alcohol-induced cirrhosis.

TABLE 10–6.—CLASSIFICATION OF LIVER BIOPSY FINDINGS RELATIVE
TO TREATMENT WITH METHOTREXATE*

Grade I	Normal, mild fatty infiltration, nuclear variability or portal inflammation
Grade II	Moderate to severe changes of Grade I
Grade III	A. Fibrous, mild
	B. Fibrous, moderate to severe
Grade IV	Cirrhosis

1. Patients with Grade I and Grade II changes may continue on methotrexate.

2. Patients with Grade IIIA changes can continue on methotrexate, but a repeat liver biopsy is suggested at 6-month intervals of continuous therapy.

3. Patients with Grade IIIB or Grade IV changes should discontinue further therapy with methotrexate.

Liver biopsies should be performed prior to initiating methotrexate therapy, during therapy at 1.5-gm cumulative dose intervals, or at 1-gm intervals or more frequently if there are significant liver abnormalities in a given patient.

Other side effects of methotrexate administration include nausea, anorexia, and fatigue. These are short-term, dose-related, and rapidly reversible. The doses should be decreased or discontinued in these patients if the side effects cause too much discomfort. Also a trial of switching between triple-dose, weekly oral dosing, or intramuscular dosing may decrease these reactions. In the older patient, reevaluating renal function may be advisable to ascertain that the patient is not having difficulties clearing the drug.

Methotrexate is a known teratogen and abortifacient and therefore pregnancy in the female patient should be strictly avoided. In the event a methotrexate patient should become pregnant, a therapeutic abortion is advised. A time period of three to four months off methotrexate should be planned prior to attempting conception for male or female patients. Oligospermia has been reported in men receiving methotrexate,[19] yet we are aware of five normal offspring of male methotrexate patients. Also, in women who received higher doses of methotrexate for choriocarcinoma and then subsequently become pregnant, the offspring were normal.

METHOTREXATE COMBINATION THERAPIES

Methotrexate has recently been combined with PUVA[11] and UVB[14] in clinical protocols. Some patients whose disease has been unresponsive to methotrexate, UVB, or PUVA alone have had good results with combinations of methotrexate and UVB or methotrexate and PUVA. Smaller amounts of methotrexate and ultraviolet light were required to clear the lesions of a majority of patients. This may be a good way to control very difficult psoriasis cases but at this time we would advocate monotherapy for two reasons: first, long-term toxicity from combined therapy is even more difficult to assess than in monotherapy and second, using only one therapy at a time allows the physician to switch from one modality to another, giving extended "rest periods" to minimize toxicity.

Methotrexate has also been used in combination with etretinate[17, 20] and colchicine[6] in patients with difficult-to-control pustular psoriasis.

OTHER SYSTEMIC AGENTS

Hydroxyurea

Hydroxyurea (Hydrea) was first proven clinically effective in psoriasis in 1970.[8] Hydroxyurea interferes with synthesis of DNA and is FDA-approved for use in malignancies only. It has been used for psoriasis on an occasional basis for selected patients, with a clinical response rate of 20%–60% and best results in pustular psoriasis.[18]

In the treatment of psoriasis, a dose of 1000–1500 mg/day for 6 to 8 weeks is recommended. Complete blood counts should be monitored weekly.

In a series of patients treated with hydroxyurea for psoriasis, 15% had adverse reactions severe enough to require stopping the drug.[12] Fever, leukopenia, thrombocytopenia, and anemia were frequent side effects. Other reactions include gastrointestinal disturbances, alopecia, macular and papular dermatitis, allergic vasculitis, fixed drug eruptions, and temporary disturbances of renal function. It is also a known teratogen.

Colchicine

Colchicine is FDA-approved for gouty arthritis and works by inhibiting chemotactic migration, blocking adhesiveness of leukocytes, stabilizing lysosomal membranes, and inhibiting mitoses. In a clinical trial of 22 patients, 50% obtained good therapeutic benefit with diminution of joint pains and best response with thin-plaque rather than thick-plaque psoriasis.[22] Three of four patients with pustular psoriasis achieved a remission within two weeks in an open study.[29]

The dosage given in these studies was in the range of 0.02 mg/kg/day given orally, three times a day. The patients were monitored by pretreatment and monthly complete blood counts, urinalyses, and SMA-12 chemistry panels, as well as bimonthly determination of B_{12} and carotene levels. No laboratory abnormalities were found but 33% complained of mild gastrointestinal symptoms such as nausea and diarrhea. Other side effects of higher-dose colchicine include bone marrow suppression, peripheral neuritis, and possible teratogenicity. There is minimal information at this time, but in the future colchicine may prove to be a useful drug, especially for pustular psoriasis, with relatively low toxicity.

Azaribine

Azaribine is a pyrimidine analogue that has clinical effect in psoriasis but also the side effects of bone marrow suppression, CNS toxicity, cardiovascular thromboses, and gastrointestinal symptoms. It was removed from the market by the FDA and remains unavailable.

Azathioprine

Azathioprine (Imuran®) is a purine analogue that is used as an immunosuppressive agent and for the chemotherapy of leukemia. It generally has been shown to be less effective than methotrexate for psoriasis, with bone marrow suppression and hepatotoxicity being its most serious side effects.[10]

Mycophenolic Acid

Mycophenolic acid is an antibiotic that inhibits nucleic acid synthesis and has activity in psoriasis. Side effects of treatment included gastrointestinal symptoms as well as an increased number of bacterial and viral infections.[10] Eli Lilly and Company voluntarily terminated its clinical trials for psoriasis in 1978.

Razoxane

Razoxane is an oral antimitotic agent that is a derivative of EDTA. In uncontrolled studies it has shown good therapeutic benefit in psoriasis without hepatotoxicity. A dose-dependent, reversible neutropenia is reported. This agent is not currently available in the United States. Recently there have been reports from Britain of myeloproliferative diseases occuring in Razoxane-treated patients.

REFERENCES

1. Ashton R., Milliward-Sadler G., White J.: Complications in MTX treatment of psoriasis with particular reference to liver fibrosis. *J. Invest. Dermatol.* 79:229–232, 1982.
2. Atherton D.J., Wells R.S., Laurent M.R., et al.: Razoxane (ICRF 159) in the treatment of psoriasis. *Br. J. Dermatol.* 102:307–317, 1980.

3. Bergstresser P.R., Schreiber S.H., Weinstein G.D.: Systemic chemotherapy of psoriasis: A national survey. *Arch. Dermatol.* 112:977–981, 1976.
4. Geronemus R., Auerbach R., Tobias H.: Liver biopsies vs. liver scans in MTX-treated patients with psoriasis. *Arch. Dermatol.* 118:649–651, 1982.
5. Halprin K.M., Fukui K., Ohkawara A.: Blood levels of MTX and the treatment of psoriasis. *Arch. Dermatol.* 103:243–249, 1971.
6. Horiguchi M., Takigawa M., Imamura S.: Treatment of generalized pustular psoriasis with MTX and colchicine. *Arch. Dermatol.* 117:760, 1981.
7. Kragballe K., Zachariae E., Zachariae H.: MTX in psoriatic arthritis: A retrospective study. *Acta Dermatol. Venereol.* 63:165–167, 1983.
8. Leavell V., Yarbro J.: Hydroxyurea, a new treatment in psoriasis. *Arch. Dermatol.* 102:144–150, 1970.
9. McCullough J.L., Weinstein G.D.: The action of cytotoxic drugs on cell proliferation in psoriasis, in Wright N., Camplejohn R. (eds.): *Psoriasis: Cell Proliferation.* Edinburgh, Churchill Livingstone, 1983, pp. 347–354.
10. McDonald C.J.: Uses of chemotherapeutic agents in psoriasis. *Pharmacol. Ther.* 14:1–24, 1981.
11. Morrison W., Khosrow Momtaz-T., Parrish J.A., et al.: Combined MTX-PUVA therapy in the treatment of psoriasis. *J. Am. Acad. Dermatol.* 6:46–51, 1982.
12. Moschella S.L., Greenwald M.A.: Psoriasis with hydroxyurea. An 18 month study of 60 patients. *Arch. Dermatol.* 107:363–368, 1973.
13. Nyfors A.: Liver biopsies from psoriatics related to MTX therapy. *Acta Pathol. Microbiol. Scand.* [A] 84:262–270, 1976.
14. Paul B.S., Khosrow Momtaz-T., Stern R.S., et al.: Combined MTX-ultraviolet B therapy in the treatment of psoriasis. *J. Am. Acad. Dermatol.* 7:758–762, 1982.
15. Rees R.B., Bennett J.H., Maibach H.I., et al.: Methotrexate for psoriasis. *Arch. Dermatol.* 95:2–11, 1967.
16. Roenigk H.H., Auerbach R., Maibach H.I., et al.: Methotrexate guidelines—revised. *J. Am. Acad. Dermatol.* 6:145–155, 1982.
17. Rosenbaum M.M., Roenigk H.H.: Treatment of generalized pustular psoriasis with etretinate and MTX. *J. Am. Acad. Dermatol.* 10:357–361, 1984.
18. Stein K., Shelly W.B., Weinberg R.A.: Hydroxyurea in the treatment of pustular psoriasis. *Br. J. Dermatol.* 85:81–85, 1971.
19. Sussman A., Leonard J.: Psoriasis, methotrexate and oligospermia. *Arch. Dermatol.* 115:215–217, 1980.
20. Vanderveen E., Ellis C.N., Campbell J.P., et al.: MTX and etretinate as concurrent therapies in severe psoriasis. *Arch. Dermatol.* 118:660–662, 1982.
21. Van Scott E.J., Auerbach R., Weinstein G.D.: Parenteral methotrexate in psoriasis. *Arch. Dermatol.* 89:550–556, 1964.
22. Wahba A., Cohen H.: Therapeutic trials with oral colchicine in psoriasis. *Acta Dermatol. Venereol.* 60:515–520, 1980.
23. Warin A.P., Landells J.W., Levine G.M., et al.: A prospective study of the effects of weekly oral methotrexate on liver biopsy: Findings in severe psoriasis. *Br. J. Dermatol.* 93:321–327, 1975.
24. Weinstein G.D., Frost P.: MTX for psoriasis: A new therapeutic schedule. *Arch. Dermatol.* 103:33–38, 1971.
25. Weinstein G.D., Goldfaden G., Frost P.: MTX: Mechanism of action on DNA synthesis in psoriasis. *Arch. Dermatol.* 104:236–243, 1971.
26. Weinstein G.D. Roenigk H., Maibach H.I., et al.: Psoriasis-liver-MTX interactions. *Arch. Dermatol.* 108:36–42, 1973.
27. Weinstein G.D., Ross P., McCullough J.L., et al.: Proliferative defects in psoriasis, in Wright N., Camplejohn R. (eds.): *Psoriasis: Cell Proliferation.* Edinburgh, Churchill Livingstone, 1983, pp. 189–208.
28. Zachariae H., Grunnet E., Sogaard H.: Liver biopsy in MTX-treated psoriatics—A reevaluation. *Acta Dermatol. Venereol.* 55:291–296, 1975.

29. Zachariae H., Kragballe K., Herlin T.: Colchicine in generalized pustular psoriasis: Clinical response and antibody dependent cytotoxicity by monocytes and neutrophils. *Arch. Dermatol. Res.* 274:327–333, 1982.
30. Zachariae H., Kragballe K., Sogaard H.: MTX induced liver cirrhosis. *Br. J. Dermatol.* 102:407–412, 1980.

11 / Synthetic Retinoids for Psoriasis

NICHOLAS J. LOWE, M.D., F.R.C.P., F.A.C.P.

VITAMIN A has been known for many years to be important for epithelial cell proliferation and differentiation.[7] It also has been used clinically to treat a number of different skin diseases, including various forms of ichthyosis, Darier's disease, and psoriasis, as well as acne. The problem that occurred with the clinical use of the high dosages of vitamin A needed to improve the skin disease was significant skin and systemic toxicity.

Recently, however, a series of synthetic derivatives of vitamin A have been synthesized and initially studied in psoriasis as well as other diseases (Plate 3).

Only one retinoid is currently available for systemic usage in the United States and that is 13-cis-retinoic acid (isotretinoin). This is extremely effective in the therapy of severe acne vulgaris. Unfortunately, it has much less effect in psoriasis, although, as will be mentioned later, it may have a role in the treatment of generalized pustular psoriasis. Additional synthetic retinoids that are currently under investigative treatment in the United States include the aromatic retinoid ethylester, also known as etretinate in the United States or Tigason in England or by the code name of Ro-10-9359. This drug was approved in 1984 in various European countries and Canada. It continues to be an investigative therapy in the United States as of August 1985.

ETRETINATE TREATMENT FOR PSORIASIS

Several studies have confirmed the efficacy of Etretinate treatment for various forms of psoriasis[1-6, 8-10, 12] (Plate 4). Most of the studies suggest that pustular and erythrodermic psoriasis are more responsive to etretinate than the chronic plaque type of psoriasis, but there is a good response in

111

plaque-type psoriasis for approximately 60% of patients.[8] However, when the drug is used alone for chronic plaque psoriasis the response to the drug is rather slow, often taking two months or longer to achieve the maximum response.

The drug is given orally, usually in a divided dose program, maximum dose being usually 1 mg/kg body weight. Significant side effects are seen in patients; Table 11–1 lists some of those side effects with their frequency as seen in a recent study of 20 patients.[6]

In Europe the drug recently has been used in combination with a series of alternative treatments, including PUVA, anthralin and topical corticosteroids.[9] It is the author's opinion that when and if the drug is approved by the FDA in this country, combination therapy will be the most practical way of using this agent. It is possible to use lower dosages of the etretinate combined with the other treatments to achieve good clinical responses in many patients. The side effects, in addition, are significantly fewer when lower dosages are used.[6]

13-CIS-RETINOIC ACID IN PSORIASIS

This drug is much less effective than etretinate for plaque and erythrodermic psoriasis. It may be used in selected patients to enhance the clinical responses to other treatments such as PUVA; however, a recent report suggested that oral 13-cis-retinoic acid is very effective in stopping the pustulation of general pustular psoriasis.[11] It seems to act as rapidly as reports

TABLE 11–1.—SIDE EFFECTS
OF ETRETINATE RO-10-9359
IN 20 PATIENTS[6]

SIGNS AND SYMPTOMS	NO. OF PATIENTS
Chapped lips	19
Dry nasal mucosa	19
Hair loss	9
Dry skin	19
Skin fragility	8
Palm/sole peeling	11
Bruising	5
Fingertip peeling	13
Thirst	7
Nosebleed	2
Sticky/clammy skin	4
Bone/joint pain	1
Irritation of eyes	3
Nail changes	4

of etretinate action in this severe and potentially dangerous stage of psoriasis. We had the opportunity to treat eight patients with generalized pustular psoriasis between 1982 and 1984. The patients had the signs of generalized pustular psoriasis with fever, malaise, chills, and leukocytosis.

13-cis-retinoic acid was given in a dose of 1.5 mg/kg per day. Within two to three days pustulation was significantly reduced or stopped completely. The drug was continued for about 4 weeks with slow reduction of dosage and start of alternative therapy (for example PUVA) to control the gradual return of plaque psoriasis.

While 13-cis-retinoic acid is not as effective as etretinate for most psoriatics, it does provide a valuable and relatively safe form of treatment for acute generalized pustular psoriasis.

OTHER SYNTHETIC RETINOIDS

Among the newer retinoids currently being evaluated in psoriasis is the arotinoid ethyl ester, which has been shown to be extremely potent in very low dosages in the therapy of psoriasis and psoriatic arthritis.[4] It does, however, seem to have the same side effects as does etretinate. There have been too few patients studied to know if it has any benefit over etretinate in the therapy of psoriasis. While the daily doses of the arotinoid (usually approximately 0.6 µg/kg body weight) are much lower than etretinate, similar side effects are seen.

Another drug that is being evaluated for effectiveness in psoriasis is a carboxylic acid metabolite of etretinate, also known as Ro-10-1670. This agent has the potential advantage of being much more rapidly excreted than etretinate. Etretinate is measurable in the body, particularly in fat tissue, as long as one year after discontinuation of dosage. Ro-10-1670, on the other hand, is rapidly excreted, usually over a few days.

One important reason to desire rapid excretion of these drugs is their potential for side effects. One particular side effect of concern is that of teratogenicity. Etretinate should not be used in women of childbearing years without contraception (and pregnancy not occur for two years after drug has last been used) because of its persistence in the body. It may be an advantage to have a more rapidly excreted drug permitting women of childbearing years to be treated under appropriate contraceptive cover and then conceive after a time off drug, should they so desire.

Again, the comparative efficacy of Ro-10-1670 with the other retinoids has not as yet been determined in a sufficiently large number of patients. Therefore, further careful clinical research is necessary into the efficacy of these alternative retinoids.

TABLE 11–2.—PSORIATIC ARTHRITIS: RESPONSES
TO RO-10-9359 THERAPY

TYPE OF SKIN PSORIASIS	JOINTS INVOLVED	IMPROVEMENT*
Erythroderma	Shoulders, hands	Yes
Erythroderma	Hips, neck, hands and feet	No
Erythroderma	Shoulders, hips and low back	No
Erythroderma	Polyarticular	Yes
Inverse	Hands	Yes
Inverse	Hands and feet	No
Plaque	Ankles and hands	Yes

*Increase in mobility with decreased pain and stiffness; less anti-inflammatory medication required.

THE EFFECTS OF SYNTHETIC RETINOIDS ON PSORIATIC ARTHROPATHY

It is interesting to note that both Ro-10-9359[6] as well as the arotinoid ethyl ester[4] were quite effective in the treatment of psoriatic arthropathy (Table 11–2). Approximately 60%–70% of patients with psoriatic arthropathy had improvement with their arthritis as witnessed by reduction in joint pain and stiffness and the need for less anti-inflammatory medication.

It may be, therefore, that this group of new drugs has potential value in other forms of inflammatory arthritis.

SUMMARY: USE OF SYNTHETIC RETINOIDS IN PSORIASIS

In the United States these agents are still under experimental investigation as of 1984. In Europe and Canada Tigason, Etretinate, (Ro-10-9359) is available. Newer synthetic retinoids include an acid metabolite of Ro-10-9359 known as Ro-10-1670, which is more rapidly excreted. A highly potent alternative retinoid is the arotinoid ethyl ester.

All of the retinoids currently studied exhibit significant side effects including dryness of the skin and mucous membranes and changes in the hair and nails. In addition, there are abnormalities of blood lipid elevation and occasional liver function test abnormalities. Some patients have developed hepatitis.

Maintenance therapy is required in nearly all patients, as a relapse of psoriasis tends to occur by eight weeks after the cessation of retinoid therapy.[6]

With Ro-10-9359 there is an overall good response or clearing in approximately 75% of patients. In addition, psoriatic arthritis improves in approximately 60% of patients.

These drugs represent a valuable advance in therapy for psoriasis and other skin diseases but they have to be used with extreme caution. All the currently available retinoids, both approved and under investigative treatment, are potent teratogens and great caution needs to be taken with contraceptive precautions in women of childbearing years. In addition, the aromatic retinoid etretinate, because of the long persistence in body tissue, should be avoided in women of childbearing years.

REFERENCES

1. Dahl B., Mollenbach K., Reymann F.: Treatment of psoriasis vulgaris with a new retinoic acid derivative RO-10–9359. *Dermatologica* 154:261–267.
2. Frederiksson T., Pettersson U.: Severe psoriasis oral therapy with a new retinoid. *Dermatologica* 157:238–244, 1978.
3. Fritsch P.: Oral retinoids in dermatology. *Int. J. Dermatol.* 20:314–329, 1981.
4. Fritsch P., Rauschmeier W., Zussner C.: Arotinoid in the treatment of psoriatic arthropathy (Abstract). *Dermatologica* 169(4):250, 1984.
5. Glazer S., Roenigk H.H.: RO-10–9359 in psoriasis. Study of effectiveness and potential heptotoxicity. *J. Invest. Dermatol.* 76:303, 1981.
6. Kaplan R.P., Russell D.H., Lowe N.J.: Etretinate therapy for psoriasis. *J. Am. Acad. Dermatol.* 8:95–102, 1983.
7. Keddie F.: Use of Vitamin A in the treatment of cutaneous diseases. *Arch. Dermatol. Syphilol.* 58:64–73, 1984.
8. Lowe N.J., Kaplan R., Breeding J.: Etretinate treatment for psoriasis inhibits epidermal ornithine decarboxylate. *J. Am. Acad. Dermatol.* 6:697–698, 1982.
9. Orfanos C.: Oral retinoids: Present status. *Br. J. Dermatol.* 103:473–482, 1980.
10. Rosenthal M.: Retinoids in der behandlung von psoriasis-arthritis. *Schweiz. Med. Wochenschr.* 109:1912–1914, 1979.
11. Sofen H., Moy R., Lowe N.J.: Isotretinoin for generalized pustular psoriasis. *Lancet* 7:4, 1984.
12. Voorhees J.J., Orfanos C.E.: Oral retinoids. *Arch. Dermatol.* 117:418–421, 1981.

12 / Psoriasis Day-Care Centers

M. ALAN MENTER, M.D.

THE CONCEPT OF day-care facilities dates back to the 1940s with the opening of psychiatric day hospitals in several cities around the world. It was not until 1958, however, that the first day hospital for patients with physical difficulties was established in Oxford, England. In 1967, Charles Grupper in Paris[5] introduced the "hospitalisation de jour" with the first true psoriasis day-care center where patients remained for treatment each day until 4 P.M. A portion of one floor of the Rothschild Hospital in Paris was developed for this purpose and contained two cubicles for application and removal of ointment, two Zimmerman ultraviolet light cabinets, two showers, four tubs, and a large room for rest and recreation.

Similarly, M.J. Woerdeman of the Department of Dermatology, Free University, Amsterdam, had assigned beds in the hospital wards in which patients were treated at night from 8 P.M. and were discharged the following morning.

In February of 1973, David Cram introduced the first day-care center in the United States at the University of California, San Francisco Hospital, to be followed shortly afterwards by the opening of Eugene Farber's psoriasis center at Stanford University Medical Center in March of 1974. Subsequently, numerous similar facilities associated with major teaching hospitals have opened in the United States, at Columbia Presbyterian Medical Center in New York, Massachusetts General Hospital in Boston, Baylor University Medical Center in Dallas, Tulane Medical Center in New Orleans, and Northwestern Medical Center in Chicago, UCLA in Los Angeles, together with similar facilities in Canada.

Harris[6] defined a day hospital as "a place in which patients spent a substantial portion of their waking time under a therapeutic regime and from which they returned to their own home or hostel to sleep at night." He estimated that the cost of running a 30-place day hospital is one-third that

116

of a 30-bed ward because it requires one nursing shift instead of three, fewer nonnursing staff, fewer items of furnishing, less expenditure on laundering, and reduced spending on food.

It has become increasingly evident, with the spiraling costs of inpatient hospital treatment in the United States, that alternative modalities of treatment such as day-care facilities will play a far greater role in treating patients with widespread psoriasis than before. While some psoriatics with severe and debilitating disease will still require inpatient hospitalization, many others may be treated adequately in day-care facilities. Likewise, at the other end of the psoriatic spectrum, the vast majority of mild to moderate cases of psoriasis can be treated adequately in the private dermatologist's office.

ESSENTIAL COMPONENTS

The facilities in a psoriasis day-care center should be similar to those found in an inpatient setting. A detailed plan of the Day Care Center at Baylor Hospital, Dallas, is shown in Fig 12–1. Full-body ultraviolet light units with adequate monitoring of UV emission are essential, together with portable and hand/foot phototherapy units. A full array of tar and anthralin preparations must be available, making the assistance of a fully trained pharmacist or pharmaceutical supply house essential. Due to the messy nature of the majority of these preparations, the facility should be furnished with stain-resistant furniture and wall coverings. Adequate ventilation, humidity, and temperature control are important, as well as sufficient plumbing capacity for regular shampooing and bathing. Bathtubs should be large and accessible enough to accommodate the many obese and arthritic patients requiring treatment. Locker rooms for storage of street clothing and personal belongings are important and separate toilet facilities for men and women necessary. A day-care lounge (Fig 12–2) with comfortable furniture, kitchen facilities (Fig 12–3), and audiovisual apparatus for lecture purposes are also needed. Optimally, a separate enclosed area for patients wishing to rest is beneficial. Adequate storage space for files, medications, and other supplies, together with separate examining areas, is also necessary.

Physical Situation

Ideally, the day-care facility should be part of, or near to, a general medical complex with an available hotel or hostel for out-of-town persons. Pa-

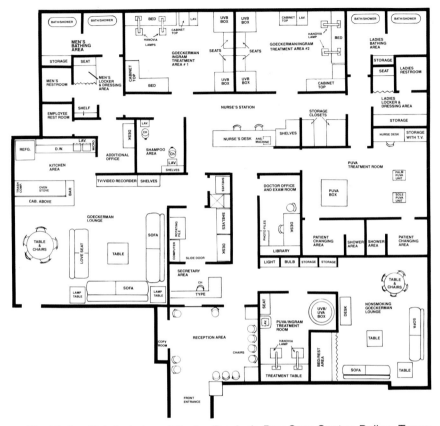

Fig 12–1.—Detailed plan of Baylor Psoriasis Day Care Center, Dallas, Texas. Total area = 2,000 sq ft.

tients with severe medical or surgical diseases or dermatologic complications might require transfer to the appropriate hospital facility.

Medical and Nursing Personnel

The presence and support of allied medical personnel is essential. A day-care facility is under the full direction of the medical director, who is responsible for the care of the patient and the supervision of other medical, nursing, and health care professionals. Each patient is fully evaluated prior to initiation of therapy. Daily examinations are performed and therapy modified as necessary. The nursing care must be provided by dermatologic

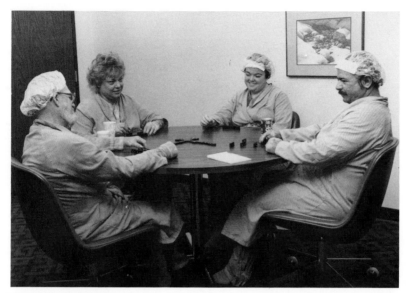

Fig 12–2.—Patients relaxing in pajamas and gowns in day care lounge after morning tar applications.

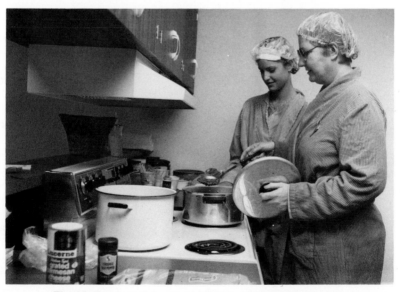

Fig 12–3.—Lunch break in kitchen off day-care lounge.

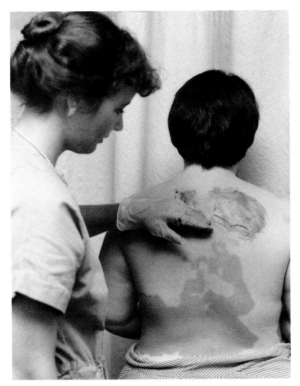

Fig 12–4.—Crude coal tar being applied to patient.

nurses who are completely trained in all aspects of light therapy, application of medications (Fig 12–4), scalp treatments (Fig 12–5), and patient education. The role of the nursing personnel in the day-care center cannot be overemphasized. The majority of patients in a day-care program are hesitant, withdrawn, and self-conscious, and a caring nurse versed in all aspects of psoriasis treatment and education plays a major role in developing a more positive outlook for the patient. Thus, regular discussion groups are led by the nursing personnel emphasizing maintenance treatment subsequent to discharge and general psoriasis and medical education for each patient.

The services of allied medical personnel are essential for the complete education and care of each patient. A good proportion of patients with severe psoriasis who enter the day-care program are obese and once clearing is obtained become highly motivated to lose weight and develop a healthier life-style. Thus, regular visits by dietitians and physical therapists are necessary, together with social workers when necessary. The help from vol-

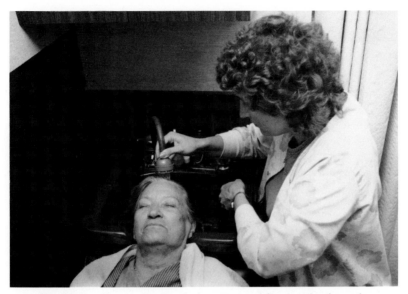

Fig 12–5.—Tar medication being removed from patient's scalp.

unteers from self-help organizations such as the various psoriasis lay groups formed in the U.K. and the U.S.A. is likewise beneficial to the patient. In order to facilitate treatment subsequent to discharge, a fully qualified pharmacist must be available, as the majority of patients have great difficulty filling tar and anthralin prescriptions at their local pharmacist.

DAY-CARE REGIMENS

Goeckerman Regimen

The need for psoriasis day-care centers grew out of a desire to more effectively administer Goeckerman treatment without the cost of hospitalization. In 1925, Goeckerman[4] developed his inpatient program for treating widespread psoriasis at the Mayo Clinic. He exposed patients daily to whole-body irradiation with ultraviolet light followed by the application of crude coal tar, and obtained total clearing within three to six weeks of treatment. Multiple variations of Goeckerman's original protocol have been proposed over the past 60 years, with the majority of treatment facilities still adhering to the tar-ultraviolet light combination.

TABLE 12–1.—GOECKERMAN REGIMEN AT BAYLOR PSORIASIS DAY CARE
CENTER, DALLAS, TEXAS

7:45 A.M.	Examination by doctor
8:00 A.M.	Exposure to ultraviolet light cabinet, plus Hanovia lamps as indicated
8:15–9:00 A.M.	Application of 2% crude coal tar (with or without 5% salicylic acid)
9:00–9:30 A.M.	Tar shampoo with application of 10–20% LCD in oil to scalp with shower cap occlusion
9:30 A.M.–12:00 noon	Rest in day-care lounge with tar occlusion under pajamas and robe. Discussion groups, counseling, psoriasis lectures, fitness and nutrition sessions
12:00 noon–1:00 P.M.	Lunch
1:00–1:30 P.M.	Oil bath with gentle removal of tar
1:30–2:00 P.M.	Repeat ultraviolet light exposure
2:00–2:30 P.M.	Application of decolorized tar (with or without occlusion) to body and scalp
3:00 P.M.	Return to home/hotel
8:00 P.M.	Reapply decolorized tar at home to body and scalp

Treatment is given six (6) days weekly with two applications of decolorized tar on Sunday.

NOTE: Anthralin ointments in increasing concentrations (0.5%–4.0%) may be substituted for resistant plaques in the Day Care Center for the afternoon application.

The routine followed by both the Dallas and San Francisco facilities is shown in Table 12–1. Treatment is given six days a week. A review of 300 patients treated in these two facilities showed an average duration of clearing of 18 days, with a 90% remission after 8 months and a 73% remission after one year, subsequent to discharge.[8] These figures parallel very closely the results obtained by Perry et al.[9] in a review of 123 patients hospitalized at the Mayo Clinic for treatment, as well as those of Armstrong et al.[1] from Columbia Presbyterian Hospital, in their series of 162 patients treated with Goeckerman therapy.

On discharge from the day-care center after a course of Goeckerman treatment, the patients are encouraged to return, where feasible, for follow-up assessment every three to six months. These patients are often extremely motivated towards follow-up care and a continued close contact with the medical and nursing personnel at the day-care center.

Ingram Regimen

In 1953, John Ingram[7] introduced the combination of anthralin and ultraviolet light for the treatment of resistant psoriasis. This is a purely outpatient regimen in which patients are exposed to increasing doses of ultraviolet light with application of anthralin pastes or ointments in increasing concentrations. As with the Goeckerman treatment, fully qualified nursing personnel are essential for application of anthralin with appropriate dressings and dosimetry of ultraviolet light. More recently, the maximum concentrations of anthralin utilized have been increased from 0.5% to 2% or even 4% in an attempt to shorten the contact time of the anthralin on the skin and minimize such side effects as irritation and staining. Excellent clearing of resistant localized plaques can be obtained in three to six weeks of purely outpatient therapy.

Combination Therapy

The addition of high-concentration anthralin to the Goeckerman regime is increasingly being utilized. Thus, anthralin ointments or pastes may be substituted for 10% liquor carbonis detergens (LCD) for resistant plaques prior to the patient's discharge each afternoon. The effects on clearing and remission rates with this modification are unknown at this stage.

BENEFITS OF PSORIASIS DAY-CARE CENTER TREATMENT

Costs

The major cause of the rapidly mounting costs of medical care must relate to in-hospital expenses. The Committee on Psoriasis of the American Academy of Dermatology[3] has published a "white paper" stressing the necessity of hospitalization facilities for patients with erythrodermic psoriasis, generalized pustular psoriasis, and disabling psoriatic arthritis. However, day-care centers are viable alternatives to costly long inpatient stays for patients who do not have such disabling disease, and have led to a marked reduction in total costs over hospitalization.

Single Unit

The placing of all equipment and facilities for the Goeckerman and Ingram regimens under one roof, together with the employment of full-time nurses, leads to a most effective course of therapy for each patient.

Patient-Patient Interaction

The majority of patients with severe psoriasis, when entering the day-care center for the first time, have little idea that there are other patients in the community with similar extensive involvement. After an initial day or two of shyness, even withdrawal from the group, most patients soon enter into the "group therapy" situation and are thus able to relate far more easily to their mutual problems. Words of encouragement from the group benefit introverted, depressed patients and a general spirit of caring, co-operation, and a desire to participate in self-help groups is frequently en-countered.

Doctor/Nurse-Patient Interaction

Seeing and examining each patient on a daily basis in the same facility enables the doctor or nurse to establish a close rapport with each individual patient and enhances their ability to help in the general education and subsequent therapy of the patient.

Clinical Trials

The combination of systemic retinoids, nonsteroidal anti-inflammatory drugs and even low-dose methotrexate with the Goeckerman or Ingram regimens is logical in attempting to improve therapy for resistant psoriatics in a day-care setting. Thus, strictly controlled therapeutic trials assessing clearing rates, remission rates, and long-term safety of these various com-binations must be pursued. The day-care center is an ideal facility for un-dertaking clinical trials of this kind.

Patient's Daily Routine

While a three-week course of Goeckerman therapy is a major commit-ment for patients, the fact that they are able to return to their families and homes each evening rather than to hospital beds must inevitably play some role in alleviating the stress and strain of therapy. Many patients also are able to return to their work place for a few hours each afternoon or early evening. For patients traveling long distances, without family or friends in the neighborhood of the day-care center, it is essential that hostel or reasonably priced hotel accommodation be available.

PROBLEMS ENCOUNTERED IN DAY-CARE FACILITIES

These have been well summarized by Chasin,[2] in relation to psychiatric day hospitals.

Irregular Attendance

Some patients habitually miss their treatments. To combat this, every effort must be made to educate patients prior to their admission to Goeckerman therapy. Due to the group nature of the day-care facility, it is essential that each patient realize the need for a structured routine and regular attendance.

Unruly, More Difficult, Behavior

Many patients are depressed when entering the treatment program and find difficulty in relating to their fellow sufferers or in following nurses' instructions. Again the role of the nursing personnel "to keep the peace" is essential and problem patients may have to be separated from the group. The female nursing personnel have to be made aware of problems they may encounter with male patients during times of application of medication. Some patients are exhibitionists and embarrass other patients: again, a firm attitude in dealing with these problems is necessary.

Non-therapeutic Attitudes

As stated by Chasin, some patients may view their attendance as a way of avoiding work or of getting away from their families. Conversely, the day-care facility may be a convenient way of having the patient looked after. Thus, it is important that the purpose of the day facility be established with the patient and family at the outset. Motivating patients to cooperate positively is a most significant factor in determining the outcome of their disease.

CRITERIA FOR ADMISSION TO GOECKERMAN THERAPY IN A DAY-CARE CENTER

The following guidelines for admission have been modified from the "white paper on hospitalization for psoriasis care."[3]

1. Severe skin damage, involving more than 25% of body surface or less than 25% but involving disabling locations such as face, hands, feet, genitalia, or skin creases, which is uncontrolled by any previous outpatient care of four weeks' or more duration.

2. Disease which is physically and/or emotionally disabling enough to limit the activities of daily living.

3. Complications from previous therapy, e.g., PUVA, anthralin, methotrexate, necessitating a change to the safer alternative of Goeckerman therapy.

4. Coexistent illnesses such as diabetes, heart disease, or arthritis that are not severe enough to warrant hospitalization and can be monitored in a day-care setting.

INSURANCE

The majority of major insurance carriers, as well as Medicare and Medicaid, have approved the day-care treatment of psoriasis, provided strict criteria are established to control admission of patients. However, continued review of these guidelines, together with postdischarge treatment guidelines, is necessary. It is encouraging to note that third-party carriers are aware of problems relating to patients traveling long distances and it is hoped that reimbursement for overnight accommodation for these patients eventually will be available, thus minimizing the need for hospitalization for convenience purposes.

CONCLUSION

There is no doubt that psoriasis day-care centers have proved to be a major advance in the treatment of severe, unresponsive psoriasis. Their goal, of providing a successful therapeutic experience for sufferers of severe psoriasis, as well as the creation of a cost-effective program in a setting totally dedicated to the physical and emotional well-being of these patients, has been met. It is logical to assume that the scope of psoriasis day-care centers will be expanded in the future to encompass other dermatologic diseases now treated by inpatient hospitalization.

REFERENCES

1. Armstrong R.B., et al.: Modified Goeckerman therapy for psoriasis. *Arch. Dermatol.* 120:313–318, 1984.
2. Chasin R.M.: Special clinic problems in day hospitalization. *Am. J. Psych.* 123:779–785, 1967.
3. Committee on Psoriasis: White paper on hospitalization for psoriasis care. *J. Am. Acad. Dermatol.* 10:842–851, 1984.
4. Goeckerman W.H.: The treatment of psoriasis. *Northwest Med.* 24:2–9, 1925.
5. Grupper C., et al.: Modifications personelles du traitment du psoriasis par la méthode de Goeckerman. *Bull. Soc. Franc. Dermatol. Syph.* 75:585–591, 1968.
6. Harris A.: Day hospitals and night hospitals in psychiatry. *Lancet* 1:729–730, 1957.
7. Ingram J.T.: Approach to psoriasis. *Br. Med. J.* 2:591–594, 1953.
8. Menter A., Cram D.: The Goeckerman regimen in two psoriasis day care centers. *J. Am. Acad. Dermatol.* 9:59–65, 1983.
9. Perry H., Soderstrom C.W., Schulze R.W.: The Goeckerman treatment of psoriasis. *Arch. Dermatol.* 98:178–182, 1968.

Comments

Nicholas J. Lowe, M.D., F.R.C.P., F.A.C.P.

These additional comments are derived from the experience of the author in establishing a skin and psoriasis treatment center at the University of California, Los Angeles School of Medicine.

It was decided to establish this unit for all the reasons itemized in the foregoing chapter. These specifically include the cost-effectiveness of day-

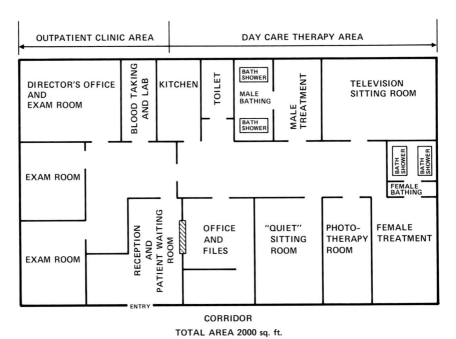

Fig 12–6.—Floor plan of Skin and Psoriasis Treatment Day Care Center, UCLA.

128

care therapy compared to inpatient hospital therapy as well as the ability to carefully train nursing staff at the treatment center in the intricacies of topical skin therapy and phototherapy. In addition, the patients are able to be treated in a more relaxed and homelike atmosphere than is possible in most inpatient hospital facilities.

The author decided to have a combined day-care center and outpatient dermatology office for staffing reasons. A floor plan of the center is shown in Fig 12–6. The advantages of this are that patients can be readily seen for follow-up visits and examinations in the adjacent outpatient office. This also leads to easier physician staffing of the center and enables the center to be utilized for varied outpatient clinical research projects.

The daily treatment outline differs slightly from that previously listed (Table 12–2). Many of the patients attending who have localized psoriasis plaques receive anthralin therapy in a short-contact mode similar to that outlined in Chapter 6. This center does not use additional ultraviolet radiation to localized areas, but relies on a single daily ultraviolet-B phototherapy session and the adjunctive use of anthralin to any resistant plaques.

In addition to providing day-care therapy, this center is utilized for brief outpatient phototherapy visits, including outpatient UVB, systemic 8-methoxypsoralen and UVA (PUVA), as well as bathwater delivery of psor-

TABLE 12–2.—USUAL REGIMEN AT SKIN AND PSORIASIS TREATMENT CENTER, UCLA

Tar and ultraviolet therapy

8:00 A.M.	Application of 2% crude coal tar in petrolatum (or equivalent), with or without 5% salicylic acid to psoriasis; tar oil or LCD in oil to unaffected skin
To 9:00 A.M.	Application of 5% tar and 5% salicylic acid in Aquaphor or Eucerin (or equivalent) to scalp, with shower cap occlusion
9:30 A.M.–12:00 noon	Rest in day-care lounges with tar occlusion under pajamas and robe. Discussion groups, counseling, psoriasis lectures
12:00 noon–2:00 P.M.	Lunch and continued rest in day-care lounges
2:00–3:00 P.M.	Ultraviolet light exposure after excess surface tar has been removed with mineral oil
3:00–3:30 P.M.	Shampoo and oil bath to gently remove all body tar
3:30–4:00 P.M.	Application of emollients
4:00 P.M.	Return to home/hotel
8:00 P.M.	Reapply purified tar at home/hotel to body and scalp (optional)

Treatment is given six (6) days weekly. The patient may apply purified tar at home on Sundays.

Anthralin therapy

Anthralin creams or ointments with increasing contact times, in increasing concentrations (0.5%–4.0%), may be used for resistant plaques for selected patients. They are applied in the afternoon and followed by removal of anthralin in shower using liquid soap.

Example: 2:00, ultraviolet light; 2:15, Anthralin applied; 2:30 to 3:15, patient showers with liquid soap to remove all anthralin.

Physician examination daily

---

alens and UVA phototherapy. Short-contact anthralin is also given during brief outpatient visits. It is possible to combine multiple treatment alternatives in this space, leading to highly efficient and effective treatment delivery.

It is the author's opinion that such a center should be considered wherever there is a significant psoriatic population needing treatment. The ideal geographical location of such a center is near a regional or teaching medical center. It is possible to use these centers for patient therapy, patient education, physician education, nursing education, and clinical research on skin diseases and therapy.

13 / Therapy of Childhood Psoriasis

Nicholas J. Lowe, M.D., F.R.C.P., F.A.C.P.

Psoriasis may present itself at any age from birth.[3] In approximately 10%–15% of patients it begins before the age of 10 years and in about 30% of patients it starts before the age of 20 years.[4] There is, therefore, a significant group of patients with psoriasis beginning in childhood.

The treatment of childhood psoriasis requires special care. Many of the treatments that we may use in adult patients should be avoided in children because of the potential for long-term and delayed toxicity.

SPECIAL PRESENTATIONS OF PSORIASIS IN CHILDREN

The first manifestation of psoriasis in some infants is the occurrence of psoriasiform dermatitis in the diaper area. This may eventually clear with therapy and the child subsequently develops more typical psoriasis later in life. The clinical presentation of psoriasis in children may also be similar to that seen in adults, with psoriasis beginning as plaques.

However, in children another form of psoriasis is quite common, that of guttate psoriasis. Psoriasis begins as the guttate form in up to 17% of all psoriasis patients (Plate 5). The guttate form may be preceded by an upper respiratory infection, commonly a streptococcal infection. It is important to exclude a focus of infection and treat any such infection promptly.

In patients in whom the psoriasis develops at an early age there appears to be an association with one of the histocompatibility antigens HL-A-17. Of further interest is that in childhood psoriasis a greater number of females than males are affected. In adults the ratio is equal in both sexes.[3]

Another form of psoriasis frequently seen in children is seborrheic psoriasis. I have already mentioned the presence of psoriasis in the diaper area; another area that may be particularly affected in children is the scalp.

DIFFERENTIAL DIAGNOSIS OF PSORIASIS IN CHILDREN

There is mainly the same differential diagnosis of psoriasis in children as in adults. There are, however, a few additional conditions to consider in children. Acrodermatitis enteropathica can occasionally mimic psoriasis, as may acropustulosis of infancy. Scabies, particularly affecting the palms and soles, can mimic pustular psoriasis. Histiocytosis X may resemble psoriasis and seborrheic dermatitis, but is usually more hemorrhagic than these diseases. Infantile pityriasis rubra pilaris is a rare papulosquamous disease that has psoriasiform features. Keratoderma blennorrhagicum occurring as part of Reiter's syndrome can produce psoriasiform lesions.

THERAPY OF CHILDHOOD PSORIASIS

Because psoriasis is a disease that may persist throughout life in variable severity, great care has to be exercised in the choice of treatment for childhood psoriasis.

Topical Therapy

TOPICAL CORTICOSTEROIDS.—While these drugs are particularly helpful in many patients with psoriasis, they must be used with great caution in childhood psoriasis. A medium-potency steroid (see Chapter 4) is the highest strength that should be allowed for childhood psoriasis. In the author's practice this is usually restricted to 0.025% triamcinolone cream or ointment or equivalent potency of steroid. The ideal is for this potency of steroid to be used in conjunction with other topical agents, such as tars and carefully supervised anthralin.

As soon as the psoriasis begins to respond to this potency of topical steroid therapy the child should receive a lower potency of steroid, for example 2.5% or 1% hydrocortisone cream or ointment.

Particular care needs to be taken with continued topical steroid application to the face and flexural areas.

In general, the higher-potency steroids should be avoided. There have been reports of the precipitation of unstable forms of psoriasis, such as generalized pustular psoriasis, on withdrawal of potent topical steroids and this may be particularly a problem with children. In addition, because of the potential effects of potent topical steroids on the pituitary-adrenal axis, these higher potency topical steroids need to be avoided in children.[1, 2]

COAL TAR PREPARATIONS.—It is this author's preference to use coal tar preparations frequently in children with psoriasis. While it is true these have relatively weak antipsoriatic action when used alone, it is my impression that they have a steroid-sparing effect and it is possible to achieve a partial improvement with the use of these agents. In addition they appear to be reasonably safe in long-term usage, there being apparently no increased incidence of skin cancer occuring in patients undergoing coal tar therapy for psoriasis. (See chapter on coal tars.)

Typical topical tar preparations are 1%, 2%, and 5% crude coal tar in petrolatum (the author rarely uses higher than 2% crude coal tar in children), 10% LCD in petrolatum or other appropriate base. Examples of some commercially available tar products include: Estar Gel, Psorigel, Baker's P and S Plus Gel, and T-Derm Tar Oil.

ANTHRALIN THERAPY.—This is occasionally useful in children with localized disease where the mother or father can be instructed to treat the child cautiously and correctly with the anthralin. (The reader is referred to Chapter 6.)

It is not practical or safe to use anthralin, however, in the young infant who is unable to remain still. In these younger patients anthralin may be smeared to the skin creases or the face and eyes and produce problems. Anthralin in children, therefore, should be restricted to the older child and should probably be used on a short-contact basis with careful instructions given and close supervision by the parent.

Children With More Severe and Resistant Psoriasis

Those patients who have failed to respond adequately to the topical therapies outlined above should, in the author's opinion, be treated as either hospital inpatients or at a day-care center.

The appropriate form of treatment is Goeckerman therapy, either alone or combined with anthralin. These treatments have stood the test of time and are considered to be relatively safe and also give the opportunity of fairly prolonged remission times.

There are children with severe and life-threatening psoriasis, such as generalized pustular psoriasis. Fortunately, this form of severe disabling, life-threatening psoriasis is extremely rare in children but when it occurs, great caution has to be exercised in selecting the type of treatment to be used.

PUVA may be used for the control of severe psoriasis in children but should not be continued for a prolonged period because of the risk of later skin cancer. Again, the guidelines outlined in Chapter 9 need to be followed.

Very occasionally, a child will have severe, uncontrolled erythroderma or generalized pustular psoriasis. In such a situation, a short course of methotrexate or systemic retinoids is occasionally indicated and justified. However, these drugs should not be continued for prolonged periods of time. Methotrexate may clearly have dangerous side effects of bone marrow suppression and longer-term liver damage.

Systemic retinoids should not be continued in children for any length of time because of potential long-term effects on the bony skeleton (retinoid-induced skeletal hyperostosis and premature epiphyseal closure) and also the potential effects of long-term lipid changes.

GENERAL FAMILY INSTRUCTIONS AND SUPPORTIVE MEASURES

It is extremely important to fully inform the parents of a child with psoriasis of the different aspects about the disease. Many parents, particularly those who have psoriasis themselves, will feel very concerned and often guilty about the fact that their child has developed psoriasis.

This will be particularly true if the child has more extensive disease. The parents should be fully counseled and encouraged by the fact that psoriasis may undergo spontaneous improvement and that good remissions may be achieved with appropriate forms of therapy. It is, however, possible that when psoriasis begins in some patients early in life the psoriasis may be more recurrent and severe.[5]

SUMMARY

It is often possible with the different forms of therapy, particularly with Goeckerman and anthralin therapy, to achieve a good improvement in the child's psoriasis. It is particularly important to take extra care in selecting antipsoriatic therapies in children because of the potential of long-term damage in the younger patient. Long-term usage of systemic agents and PUVA is to be avoided whenever possible.

REFERENCES

1. Boxley J.D., Dawber R.P.R., Summerly R.: Generalized pustular psoriasis on withdrawal of clobetasol propionate ointment. *Br. Med. J.* 2:255–256, 1975.

2. Carruthers J.A., August P.J., Stoughton R.C.: Observations on the systemic effect of topical clobetasol propionate. *Br. Med. J.* 4:203–204, 1975.
3. Farber E.M., Carlsen R.A.: Psoriasis in childhood. *California Med.* 105:415–420, 1966.
4. Farber E.M., Nall M.L.: The natural history of psoriasis in 5,600 patients. *Dermatologica* 148:1–18, 1974.
5. Loeffel E.D.: Psoriasis in adolescence, in Solomon Y.M., Esterly N.B., Loeffel E.D. (eds.): *Adolescent Dermatology.* Philadelphia, W.B. Saunders, 1978, pp. 143–162.
6. Pittelco M.R., Pery H.O., Mueller S.A.: Skin cancer in patients undergoing a coal tar therapy for psoriasis. *J. Int. Dermatol.* 77:181–185, 1981.

14 / Scalp Psoriasis: Practical Aspects of Therapy

Nicholas J. Lowe, M.D., F.R.C.P., F.A.C.P.

PSORIASIS OF the scalp is often a major problem for the patient. It can be extremely difficult to treat. Scalp psoriasis is often very socially embarassing for the patient and very challenging for the physician to manage.

The incidence of scalp involvement may not be accurately known but it probably occurs in at least 50% of psoriasis patients from time to time. The scalp may be the only area involved in some patients; in other patients, extensive psoriasis may occur on other parts of the body but the scalp spared. The severity of the scalp psoriasis may also vary, ranging from a fine, diffuse scale to thickened, armor-like plaques of scale affecting the entire scalp (Plate 6).

HISTOPATHOLOGY OF SCALP PSORIASIS

The histologic features of psoriasis include parakeratosis, reduced or absent granular cell layer, and regular epidermal acanthosis with elongation of the rete pegs. There are usually collections of polymorphonuclear leukocytes and lymphocytes in the epidermis. When they are sufficiently large to be seen as abscesses they are known as Munro microabscesses. The dermal capillaries are often tortuous and inflammatory cell infiltrate is present in the upper dermis.[1]

The major clinical differential diagnosis of scalp psoriasis is that of seborrheic dermatitis. There are often great similarities in the histopathology of seborrheic dermatitis and psoriasis. If there is spongiosis or spongiatic vesicles, then more likely it favors seborrheic dermatitis. The features favoring psoriasis include prominent parakeratosis, positive PAS inclusions in the keratinocytes and a regular acanthosis.

136

There is often clinical and histopathologic overlap and diagnostic confusion between psoriasis and seborrheic dermatitis. Hair follicle kinetics are not increased in psoriasis.[2, 16] Psoriasis usually does not cause alopecia, although a diffuse alopecia may occur as a telogen effluvium as a result of widespread skin disease.

Hair shaft abnormalities in psoriasis have been described.[19]

From the practical point of view the treatments of both of these conditions are very similar, although seborrheic dermatitis, in this author's opinion, responds more readily than does scalp psoriasis, which often becomes more stubborn and resistant to topical therapy.

PRACTICAL ASPECTS OF THERAPY

It is convenient to separate the different severities of scalp psoriasis, as they often require different forms of therapy.

MILD DIFFUSE SCALP PSORIASIS.—This is the form which is most readily confused with seborrheic dermatitis. This form of scalp psoriasis often responds well to regular shampooing with tar- and salicylic acid-containing preparations. In addition, the use of phenol and saline solutions at night and medium-potency topical corticosteroid lotions during the day is often extremely useful and adequate to control this form of scalp psoriasis.

LOCALIZED PLAQUE FORM OF SCALP PSORIASIS.—Localized small plaques of psoriasis within the scalp, again, often respond to local forms of tar- and salicylic acid-containing preparations.

In the author's opinion, this form of localized scalp psoriasis also responds extremely well to careful intralesional dermal injections of triamcinolone. The author usually restricts the concentration to 5 mg per cc and care is taken not to inject more than a total of 1 cc at each office visit. Ideally this treatment should not be repeated more frequently than once every four to six weeks. Care also should be taken to avoid overly repetitive use of this treatment because it may lead to significant scalp atrophy and the possibility of more widespread systemic effects of the corticosteroid. Between these treatments, the use of the therapies outlined above for milder forms of scalp psoriasis should be continued as these may help to reduce the incidence of relapse of the disease.

EXTENSIVE, SEVERE SCALP PSORIASIS.—The treatment of this form of psoriasis is particularly difficult and challenges the dermatologist.

It is often necessary to change from one form of therapy to another in an attempt to prevent resistance to therapy.

It is necessary to carefully choose the therapy if you are attempting to treat the patient at home, simply because the messy occlusive ointments are often extremely difficult for the patient to use at home as they are cosmetically unattractive and there is great difficulty of removal.

Home Treatment

For practical home treatment, the author uses the following preparations.

At night the patient applies a tar- and salicylic acid-containing preparation. This can either be one of the tar and salicylic acid gels, for example Bakers P and S Plus Gel, or a lotion, for example Neutrogena Tar and Salicylic Acid Scalp Lotion. Another alternative is to combine a tar gel (Estargel, Psorigel) with salicylic acid gel (for example, Keralyt Gel). These preparations are rubbed well into the scalp at night and may be covered with a plastic or paper shower cap. In the morning, the patient wets the scalp thoroughly in a shower or basin and rubs in a tar-containing shampoo, wrapping the scalp in a damp, warm towel. This is left on the scalp for approximately 15 minutes—the patient can have a cup of coffee or read during this time. The patient then returns to the shower and removes this initial shampoo, then repeats the shampooing until the nocturnal cream or gel preparations have been removed.

Once during the day, if required, the scalp can be treated with a single application of a high-potency corticosteroid lotion (Lidex Solution, Diprosone Lotion).

If the response to this therapy is slow, an anthralin preparation can be used additionally for fifteen minutes before showering as a form of short-contact anthralin scalp therapy. In the author's experience 1% Dithrocream is practical as it can be easily washed out of the scalp. Another alternative is to have the pharmacist formulate anthralin 1% in a propylene glycol vehicle. Great care must be taken to instruct the patient not to get anthralin in the eyes and to thoroughly wash the anthralin from the scalp.

Day-Care or Hospital Scalp Treatment

When the psoriasis is being treated on an inpatient basis or at a day-care center for psoriasis elsewhere, then other preparations can be used for scalp therapy. For example, during the stay at a day-care center or overnight in the hospital it is possible to use 5% crude coal tar and 5% or 10% salicylic acid in an ointment base. Liquor carbonis detergens may be substituted for crude coal tar; oil of cade is another useful preparation.

PREPARATIONS USEFUL FOR TREATING SCALP PSORIASIS

Phenol and Saline Solution

This has been used for some years in the therapy of scalp psoriasis. There is a relative lack of understanding about the precise pharmacologic action of this mixture. In general, it is only useful for relatively mild psoriasis or previously severe forms of scalp psoriasis that have already been treated with other, more potent forms of active therapy. It is usually used overnight and is readily removed by shampooing the following morning.

Salicylic Acid Preparations

Salicyclic acid is extremely helpful in many scaling skin diseases. The precise mechanism of action is not known but may involve a keratolytic effect on stratum corneum, leading to more ready desquamation and stratum corneum shedding. Salicylic acid may be incorporated into lotion, gel or ointment vehicles or may be included with other active agents, such as coal tars or anthralin. The usual concentration is between 2% and 10%. Some patients note irritation and itching with the higher concentrations. Caution is required in children because excessive topical application can result in skin absorption and systemic effects of the salicylic acid. Useful salicylic acid containing preparations in the U.S. include: Keralyt Gel, Bakers P & S Plus Gel, and Neutrogena Tar and Salicylic Acid lotion.

Topical Corticosteroids

Probably the most frequently used topical treatments for scalp psoriasis are corticosteroids in alcohol solutions, lotions, or gels. In the author's experience these are not particularly effective when used alone in thick, recalcitrant scalp psoriasis. They are more useful and effective in milder forms of scalp psoriasis and also in scalp psoriasis that has been improved with other forms of therapy.

One general problem with extensive use of topical corticosteroids in psoriasis is that a rapid relapse may occur when the steroid is stopped. Skin atrophy can occur with prolonged use. There is also a concern in childhood psoriatics of pituitary-adrenal axis suppression after excessive long-term topical steroid application.

Table 14–1 lists some of the corticosteroid preparations suitable for the treatment of scalp psoriasis available in the United States.

Coal Tar Preparations

Coal tars have been used to treat several different skin diseases for many years. Goeckerman in 1925 introduced the concept of combining ultraviolet radiation and coal tar.[5] Many subsequent studies have been conducted to further evaluate the use of coal tars with or without ultraviolet light in the treatment of psoriasis. Some studies have indicated that coal tars are useful agents alone[3]; others have confirmed the usefulness of coal tars with ultraviolet radiation.[11-13] We recently showed that a topical tar oil had a definite antipsoriatic effect, superior to the oil base alone when used on extensor psoriasis of the legs without ultraviolet radiation.[11]

TABLE 14–1.—SOME PREPARATIONS
FOR TREATING SCALP PSORIASIS
AVAILABLE IN THE UNITED STATES

Steroid preparations
Aristocort Lotion
Cordran Lotion
Diprosone Lotion
Diprosone Gel Aerosol
Lidex Solution
Synalar Lotion
Lidex Gel
Valisone Lotion
Purified tar preparations
Baker's P and S Plus Gel
Estar Tar Gel
Fototar Tar Cream
Psorigel
T-Derm Tar Oil
T-Derm Tar and Salicylic Acid Scalp Lotion
Salicylic acid preparations
Keralyt Gel
Other preparations
P and S Liquid

The precise mechanism of pharmacologic action of coal tars on psoriasis is not known. Several possible mechanisms may be involved. When coal tars are applied to normal skin there is an early suppression of epidermal DNA synthesis[9, 18] followed by a proliferative response. If the treatment is continued for as long as 40 days there is a subsequent cytostatic effect of the tars, with resultant epidermal thinning.[7] In addition, many clinicians consider that coal tars have anti-inflammatory, as well as antipruritic, properties.

Coal tars may be used in the treatment of scalp psoriasis, either alone or combined with salicylic acid preparations. There are various vehicles that may be used, ranging from creams and ointments to more practical scalp treatment vehicles such as gels and oils.

Crude coal tar is often extremely difficult for patients to use at home, although it is an extremely useful and effective therapy for inpatient or day-care center treatment. Between 2% and 5% crude coal tar plus 5%–10% salicylic acid may be incorporated in a petrolatum vehicle, usually applied overnight.

A further preparation that may be used is a combination of oil of cade 6%, precipitated sulfur 2%, and emulsifying ointment to 100%. This, again, is applied overnight and removed as described for the tar ointments.

Liquor carbonis detergens, 5%–15%, may be substituted for crude coal tar and in general is less messy and more usable. No well-controlled study has been conducted to determine whether it is as active therapeutically as crude coal tar.

Purified tar preparations are valuable for the treatment of scalp psoriasis and are more easily used on an outpatient basis. Purified tar gels were shown to be effective in a topical scalp psoriasis study reported recently.[6]

Table 14–1 lists some purified tar products useful for treating scalp psoriasis that are available in the U.S.

Anthralin Preparations

Anthralin has been used for many years as an antipsoriatic[4, 17] and is a useful therapy for some patients with scalp psoriasis, but additional care has to be taken in its usage to avoid unwanted eye contamination and irritation. Different vehicle formulations may be used, but again, the same problems may occur if ointment vehicles are used as when coal tar ointments are used, there being great difficulty in removing the ointment vehicles with appropriate scalp shampooing. Anthralin creams are more easily applied and removed from scalp psoriasis. Anthralin probably has to be used in concentrations above 0.1% to be effective in most situations.[8]

A recent modification of anthralin for skin psoriasis, where higher concentrations remain on the skin for a brief period of time, is the so-called short-contact therapy of anthralin.[15] This has received significant attention as a body psoriasis treatment. Anthralin 0.5% or 1% cream applied to the scalp and washed out after 15 minutes is very useful for some patients.

The major problems of anthralin therapy are skin irritation and staining. Its use needs to be closely monitored; in particular, any excess should be removed from the skin and no contact with the eyes must be allowed. This is often more achievable using the short-contact treatment approach, although very careful shampooing is necessary.

Shampoo Preparations

Shampoo preparations may contain a variety of active ingredients. The most common ingredients for shampoos used for scalp psoriasis include coal tars and salicylic acid, as well as sulfur and selenium.

Coal tar shampoos have probably been the most successful in the treatment of scalp psoriasis. A recent attempt was made to evaluate the biologic and potential pharmacologic activity of these products using the epidermal DNA synthesis suppression assay.[9] In these studies we found that different coal-tar containing shampoos showed marked variability in their ability to suppress DNA synthesis. This assay has been shown to correlate with antipsoriatic effectiveness of other topical agents.[10]

A further study of the treatment of scalp psoriasis also confirmed the value of tar-containing shampoo, compared to a non-tar-containing shampoo in the maintenance therapy of psoriasis.[6] These workers found that psoriasis patients remained in remission for a longer period of time if they were using tar shampoo for their scalp psoriasis rather than a non-tar-containing shampoo.[6]

Other shampoos having some effectiveness against mild to moderate scalp psoriasis contain salicylic acid, sulfur, or selenium as therapeutic agents. To the author's knowledge no direct comparison has been made of these diffferent shampoo ingredients and there is a lack of information on the efficacy of different coal tar shampoos.

My own preference for the patient with scalp psoriasis is to advise the use of a coal tar-containing shampoo as frequently as necessary. Patients who have active scalp psoriasis should use the shampoo on a daily basis. I usually suggest wetting the scalp with warm water, rubbing the tar-containing shampoo well into the scalp, and then wrapping a warm, damp towel around the scalp for 15 minutes. The patient then showers and repeats the procedure. It is to be anticipated that any active therapeutic agents from the tar shampoo will have the opportunity to penetrate the scalp skin and produce a pharmacologic effect.

SCALP PSORIASIS RESPONSE TO SYSTEMIC THERAPY

Clearly, any systemic therapy being used to control the psoriasis is likely to improve scalp psoriasis. This is true for systemic methotrexate and also for systemic synthetic retinoids such as etretinate, which is extremely valuable in the treatment of psoriasis.

I have recently had the opportunity to treat some patients with an alternative synthetic retinoid, Accutane (13-cis-retinoic acid). This is a most effective antiacne therapy, but occasionally is useful for some psoriasis patients. The response rate to Accutane, however, is not nearly as good in psoriasis as the response to etretinate (personal observations). If, however, thick scalp psoriasis resistant to topical therapy is present, then a four-to-eight-week course of oral Accutane (1 mg/kg body weight) plus continued topical therapy is useful in reducing the thickness of the scale and increasing the response rate. It should be noted that the systemic retinoids have significant side effects; in particular, patients will develop severe mucocutaneous drying. In addition, careful fasting blood evaluations need to be made, particularly noting changes in serum lipid patterns. Women of childbearing years have to be on an effective form of contraception as these agents are teratogens. Long-term usage may lead to skeletal changes of hyperostosis.

A further agent that has been suggested as being effective in some patients with psoriasis is ketoconazole. This drug was reported by Rosenberg as being effective in some patients with psoriasis;[14] the theoretical reason for this effectiveness being a depletion of surface yeast contaminants. The yeast contaminants are thought to activate the complement cascade in psoriasis skin leading to leukocyte chemotaxis.[14] These findings remain to be confirmed by others; however, with chronic scalp psoriasis resistant to other therapy, a course of ketoconazole may be justified. Again, caution is needed because of potential systemic side effects, particularly of hepatotoxicity. A careful history to rule out hepatic disease in the patient is most important as well as blood examinations including hepatic function tests.

Finally, in those patients with significant baldness or very short hair and the presence of scalp psoriasis the use of psoralen and UVA (PUVA) photochemotherapy will result in the improvement of psoriasis. In my experience PUVA is largely of no help for those patients who have significant hair growth, owing to ultraviolet shielding.

SUMMARY

The scalp is frequently involved in psoriasis patients and poses a therapeutic challenge to the patient and physician. It is often necessary to use combinations of topical treatment, as well as to change the topical therapy regularly, to achieve and maintain good control of scalp psoriasis. In severe, recalcitrant, socially incapacitating scalp psoriasis, it may be necessary to consider using systemic therapy with appropriate precautions.

REFERENCES

1. Braun-Falco O., Heilgemeir G.P., Lincke-Plewig H.: Histologische differentialdiagnose von vulgaris und seborrhoischen. Ekzem des kapillitium. *Hautarzt* 30(1):478–483, 1979.
2. Comaish S.: Autoradiographic studies of hair growth in various dermatoses. *Br. J. Derm.* 81:283–288, 1969.
3. Ellis C.C., Wooldrige W.E., Weiss R.S.: The treatment of psoriasis with liquor carbonis detergens. *J. Int. Dermatol.* 10:455–459, 1948.
4. Galewsky: Uber Cignolin, ein Ersatzpraparat des chryosarbins. *Dermatol. Wschnschr.* 6:113–115, 1916.
5. Goeckerman W.H.: The treatment of psoriasis. *Northwest Med.* 24:229–331, 1925.
6. Langner A., Wolska H., Hebborn P.: Treatment of psoriasis of the scalp with coal tar gel and shampoo preparations. *Cutis* 32:290–296, 1983.
7. Lavker R.M., Grove G.R., Kligman A.M.: The atrophogenic effect of crude coal tar on human epidermis. *Br. J. Dermatol.* 105:77–82, 1981.
8. Lowe N.J., Breeding J.: Anthralin: Different concentrations effects on epidermal DNA synthesis in mice and clinical responses in human psoriasis. *Arch. Dermatol.* 117:698–700, 1981.
9. Lowe N.J., Wortzman M.S., Breeding J.: Evaluation of efficacy of a new coal extract and coal tar shampoos by epidermal DNA synthesis suppression assay. *Arch. Dermatol.* 118:487–489, 1982.
10. Lowe N.J., Stoughton R.B., McCullough J.L., et al.: Topical drug effects on normal and proliferating epidermal cell models. *Arch. Dermatol.* 117:394–398, 1981.
11. Lowe N.J., Wortzman M.S., Breeding J., et al.: Coal tar phototherapy for psoriasis reevaluated. *J. Am. Acad. Dermatol.* 8:781–789, 1983.
12. Marsico A.R., Eaglstein W.H., Weinstein G.D.: Ultraviolet light and tar in the Goeckerman treatment of psoriasis. *Arch. Dermatol.* 112:1249–1250, 1976.
13. Perry H.O., Soderstrom C.W., Schultze R.W.: The Goeckerman treatment of psoriasis. *Arch. Dermatol.* 98:178–182, 1968.
14. Rosenberg E.W., Belew P.W.: Role of microbial factors in psoriasis, in Farber E.M., Lox A.J.: *Proceedings: The Third International Symposium.* New York, Grune and Stratton, 1982, pp. 343–344.
15. Runne U., Kunze J.: Short duration therapy with Dithranol for psoriasis. *Br. J. Dermatol.* 106:135–139, 1982.
16. Sharad B., Marks R.: Hair follicle kinetics in psoriasis. *Br. J. Dermatol.* 94:7–12, 1976.
17. Squire B.: Chrysophonic acid ointment. *Pharm. J. Trans.* 36:489–490, 1876.
18. Walter J.F., Stoughton R.B., De Quoy P.R.: Suppression of epidermal DNA synthesis by ultraviolet light, coal tar and anthralin. *Br. J. Dermatol.* 99:89–96, 1978.
19. Wyatt E., Bottoms E., Comaish S.: Abnormal hair shafts in psoriasis in scanning electron microscopy. *Br. J. Dermatol.* 87:368–373, 1972.

15 / Therapy of Pustular Psoriasis

Nicholas J. Lowe, M.D., F.R.C.P, F.A.C.P.

WHILE THE HISTOPATHOLOGY of psoriasis is often characterized by an accumulation of polymorphonuclear leukocytes in the epidermis, there are no obvious clinical pustules present in most patients with psoriasis vulgaris. However, there are situations when clinically obvious pustules appear. These are the localized types of pustular psoriasis—usually affecting the palms and soles. Another type is that of generalized pustular psoriasis, a severe and occasionally fatal form of psoriasis characterized by generalized pustules and systemic symptoms.

The remainder of this chapter will deal with the treatment of firstly localized pustular psoriasis and secondly generalized pustular psoriasis. These types of psoriasis are often extremely challenging to the physician, requiring different therapeutic approaches than are used for the treatment of the other types of psoriasis.

CLINICAL PATTERNS OF PUSTULAR PSORIASIS

Pustular psoriasis, as noted, may be either localized or generalized.

Localized pustular psoriasis (Plate 7) usually affects the palms and soles; it may also affect the nail beds. It may be known as palmar-plantar pustular psoriasis, although there are several other names. A variant type has been called acrodermatitis continua of Hallopeau.[3] Other types of this disease occur as part of Reiter's syndrome and are also known as keratoderma blennorrhagica.

These localized forms of pustular psoriasis may arise without any evidence of psoriasis vulgaris elsewhere; however, in the author's opinion, areas of classical psoriasis on other parts of the body are seen with sufficient frequency in association with localized pustular psoriasis of the palms and soles that it is likely that this is a variant form of psoriasis vulgaris. This is classically a disease of middle age or the elderly and is quite uncommon in children.

The disease usually starts as symmetrical areas of involvement on the palms or the soles. There is usually a mixture of white and brown pustules with associated erythema and often a thick, indolent scale. The pustules are usually quite discrete, approximately 5 mm in diameter. While there is usually no well-defined plaque present on the palms and soles, the disease is quite frequently found in association with localized plaques of psoriasis vulgaris elsewhere on the body. The etiology is unknown, as is the etiology of psoriasis vulgaris.

Generalized pustular psoriasis is almost always preceded by the more common type of psoriasis, either the plaque or erythrodermic phase of the disease.

Generalized pustular psoriasis (Plate 8) was originally described by Leopold Von Zumbusch.[13] He described the occurrence of generalized pustulation on an erythematous base in association with systemic symptoms of fever, malaise, and rigors. His original two cases were familial. A similar entity previously described under the term impetigo herpetiformis was probably generalized pustular psoriasis arising during pregnancy.[4]

It is possible for patients with generalized pustular psoriasis to be severely ill and have significant fluid and electrolyte imbalance. In addition they respond quite differently and often dramatically to different forms of therapy.

THERAPY OF LOCALIZED PUSTULAR PSORIASIS

The therapy of localized pustular psoriasis may be divided into topical therapy and systemic therapy. A combination of systemic and local therapy using oral methoxsalen and local UVA (PUVA) is a further alternative.

Topical Therapy

The most frequently used topical therapeutic agents for localized pustular psoriasis, as with other forms of psoriasis, are the higher-potency topical corticosteroids. These agents are covered in detail in Chapter 4.

There are special ways of using topical corticosteroids in localized palmar-plantar psoriasis. In view of the thickness of the stratum corneum in this disease and the resistance to therapy, even when potent topical corticosteroids are used they need often to be used under plastic occlusion to enhance skin penetration. In the author's experience the most effective way of using topical corticosteroids in localized pustular psoriasis is to use an ointment base rather than a cream base. The steroid ointment is applied in the evening, usually one hour before bed, and the patient wears either plastic disposable gloves or a plastic bag on the feet covered with socks.

It is often unpleasant or uncomfortable for patients to have to wear the plastic coverage in bed at night. It is, however, often possible for them to keep the plastic occlusion on for one hour prior to bed, insuring sufficient penetration of the corticosteroid.

Inevitably, all of the side effects of topical corticosteroids have to be observed. One of these is skin atrophy: often on the palms and soles painful fissures of the psoriasis become a problem to the patient. Again, in the author's experience, when this painful fissuring occurs it is often necessary to stop using the corticosteroid preparations as they most certainly inhibit re-epithelialization of these areas.

With dry, fissured psoriasis it is often useful to combine a medium to lower potency topical corticosteroid with a more emollient vehicle containing ten percent urea. The reader is referred to Chapter 4 for further information on topical corticosteroids in psoriasis. Potent topical corticosteroids may occasionally lead to more severe pustulation.

Other topical agents that are often useful as adjunctive therapies with the corticosteroid are anthralin and coal tars. This author often will suggest the use of a topical corticosteroid once daily and a before-bed application of a coal tar preparation. When the palmar-plantar psoriasis is extremely hyperkeratotic, the patient may use a coal tar preparation also containing a 5% or 10% concentration of salicylic acid. Again, all the different coal tar preparations are separately covered in Chapter 5 and the reader is referred there for further information.

Anthralin is often useful in this condition and may be used for brief periods of time in a short-contact mode of therapy. This therapeutic agent is fully discussed in Chapter 6. For practical purposes, in plamar-plantar psoriasis the author prefers anthralin in an ointment base (either one of the commercially available anthralin ointments or a formulation of anthralin in petrolatum). The patient may need to cover the anthralin for 30 minutes to an hour with plastic occlusion with much less risk of skin irritation on the palms and soles than on other skin sites.

Again, a single application of anthralin and a single application of topical corticosteroid is often an effective way of achieving good initial response. The topical corticosteroid is then discontinued and the patient continues with anthralin therapy.

PUVA Phototherapy

A PUVA phototherapy regimen may use either topical[12] or oral 8-meth-oxypsoralen.[6] The advantages and disadvantages of topical versus systemic psoralens are fully covered in Chapter 9. For practical purposes the author prefers the use of 0.1% 8-methoxypsoralen in an ointment base (petrolatum). This may be applied for one hour under plastic occlusion prior to using local UVA hand and foot units.

It is critical to carefully regulate the amount of ultraviolet used for this topical therapy, as only approximately one tenth of the amount of UVA is required with topical psoralens as with systemic psoralens to produce a phototoxic response. Practically, this means that using topical 0.1% 8-methoxypsoralen ointment, initial treatments are usually 0.1–0.3 J/sq cm of UVA. Later during therapy the concentration of 8-methoxypsoralen may be increased to 0.5% or 1%.

If the patient is receiving systemic psoralen for whole-body psoriasis, it is possible after the whole-body treatment in an upright PUVA unit to give them additional UVA to the palms and soles. This is often an extremely valuable adjunctive therapy if there is resistant psoriasis in these areas.

Other topical therapies that have been discussed elsewhere in this book include the liberal use of emollients, salicylic acid, and urea-containing preparations. These often are extremely important to use in conjunction with other forms of topical and systemic therapy.

Systemic Therapy For Localized Palmar-Plantar Psoriasis

SYNTHETIC RETINOIDS.—The synthetic retinoids are a major advance in the treatment of both localized as well as generalized pustular psoriasis. Some dermatologists feel that these are a treatment of first choice for these two conditions.[11]

The synthetic retinoid most investigated in both Europe and in the United States for psoriasis therapy is Etretinate, also known as RO-10-9359 and Tigason in Europe. The retinoids as a group of drugs are discussed in fuller detail in Chapter 11.

It has been well described that localized pustular psoriasis responds extremely well to etretinate. Some of the author's patients with psoriasis vulgaris elsewhere also had localized palmar-plantar pustular psoriasis. These palmar-plantar lesions responded rapidly to the start of therapy with etretinate. The average dose required initially is between 0.5 mg and 1 mg per kg body weight. With localized pustular psoriasis it is anticipated that a maximum response will be seen by approximately 4 to 6 weeks of therapy. All of the important factors concerning toxicity and side effects of these drugs need to be considered carefully.

One particular warning with these drugs is to avoid therapy in women who are likely to become pregnant. These drugs are potent teratogens. The other side effects are covered fully in Chapter 11.

METHOTREXATE THERAPY.—Systemic antimetabolites have been used for some time in the therapy of psoriasis vulgaris. Chapter 10 reviews in detail the use of these different chemotherapeutic agents in the therapy of psoriasis vulgaris.

It is occasionally necessary to consider the use of methotrexate in the management of a person with severe, recalcitrant, disabling, localized palmar-plantar psoriasis.

The same dosage schedule is usually used as with more generalized forms of psoriasis. In the author's experience methotrexate is best used as a single weekly dosage. If the patient is reliable and gets no nausea from the drug then the methotrexate may be given orally. If it is an unreliable patient or if there is significant nausea, then the methotrexate may be delivered once weekly by intramuscular injection.

The appropriate patient selection and pretreatment evaluations required prior to considering methotrexate are covered in detail in Chapter 10.

In the author's experience systemic methotrexate is often valuable for a small group of patients with localized resistant palmar-plantar pustular psoriasis. It is not usually as effective as etretinate. It takes often many weeks for the methotrexate to be effective and there are patients whose palmar-plantar psoriasis is methotrexate-resistant.

Another drug that is less effective is hydroxyurea. Again, this is covered in detail in Chapter 10.

A further agent described as being effective in some patients with localized palmar-plantar pustular psoriasis is colchicine.[10] In this author's experience this drug has failed to show significant benefit in most patients.

SUMMARY: LOCALIZED PUSTULAR PSORIASIS OF THE PALMS AND SOLES

The therapy of this variant form of psoriasis is often extremely challenging. In the author's experience the more potent topical steroids and anthralin are often required. Valuable forms of therapy include local 8-methoxypsoralen and UVA phototherapy. Synthetic retinoids are an extremely valuable therapy in those patients unresponsive to conventional topical therapy or PUVA phototherapy. Table 15–1 summarizes the types of therapy available for localized pustular psoriasis.

TABLE 15–1.—SUMMARY OF THERAPEUTIC
OPTIONS FOR LOCALIZED PUSTULAR PSORIASIS

Topical Therapy
    Topical steroids (potent), with and without occlusion
    Coal tar and salicylic acid ointments
    Anthralin
    Intralesional steroids (Kenalog, 5–10 mg/cc)
Systemic Therapy
    Methotrexate
    Systemic retinoids

GENERALIZED PUSTULAR PSORIASIS THERAPY

General Comments

In the author's experience the wisest choice for patients with generalized pustular psoriasis is for them to be admitted to an acute care or dermatology hospital ward. This is important because the patients are occasionally acutely ill and there have been fatalities described of patients with generalized pustular psoriasis. Occasionally in generalized pustular psoriasis occuring during pregnancy it may be necessary to terminate the pregnancy.

General Nursing Measures

It is important that the patient be nursed in bed, with care and attention paid to temperature regulation plus fluid and electrolyte balance. Adequate fluid intake must be maintained. It is possible when large areas of the body are involved with generalized pustulation that there is a most ineffective skin barrier present and large amounts of fluid and electrolytes may be lost through the skin.

General Topical Measures

Bland emollients should be used routinely, applied 3–4 times daily, in an attempt to reduce the skin discomfort as well as to inhibit some of the percutaneous fluid and electrolyte loss often seen with this condition. If the patient has been applying large amounts of potent topical steroids then these should be continued during the acute pustular phase of the reaction. At a later stage, when the patient is more stable, these agents can be slowly reduced in potency and withdrawn.

In general, coal tars, anthralin, and salicylic acid preparations, which are so valuable in other forms of psoriasis, should be avoided in generalized pustular psoriasis. They sometimes worsen or precipitate the problem.

SYSTEMIC THERAPY

Synthetic Retinoids

In the author's experience, the drugs of choice now in the management of acute generalized pustular psoriasis are the synthetic retinoids. Both etretinate as well as isotretinoin (13-cis-retinoic acid) have been described as producing a rapid response and cessation of pustules in this potentially severe problem.

Patients with generalized pustular psoriasis of the Von Zumbusch type recently have been studied at the author's institution under his care.[8] They were treated with bed rest and 13-cis-retinoic acid in a dosage of 1.5 mg/ kg body weight. All patients had large total body surface areas of involvement with additional symptoms of fever and leukocytosis.

The pustules and febrile episodes began improving by the second or third day of 13-cis-retinoic acid therapy and had cleared completely after five days of therapy in all patients. After between seven and 14 days of therapy the dosage was slowly decreased. In some patients a local recurrence of pustules occurred with this lowered dosage. These patients again responded to an increased dosage of oral 13-cis-retinoic acid, suggesting a definite direct pharmacologic action of this agent on the pustulation. In all of the patients with pustular psoriasis the response to 13-cis-retinoic acid was found to be dose-dependent. Plate 9 shows a typical patient response.

Other workers have described a good and rapid response to etretinate[7] and it is likely that both these retinoids are extremely important in the management of this severe phase of psoriasis. It should be stressed that for the continued management of the psoriasis once the pustulation has resolved, etretinate is far superior to 13-cis-retinoic acid (N.J. Lowe, et al., unpublished observations).

PUVA Photochemotherapy

PUVA photochemotherapy is often extremely useful in the management of generalized pustular psoriasis; however, in the author's experience it is wise to allow the patient to partially recover from the severe stage of the condition prior to starting PUVA therapy. Some of the author's patients whose generalized pustulation was stopped with oral 13-cis-retinoic acid were subsequently started on oral PUVA therapy. The 13-cis-retinoic acid was then slowly withdrawn in those patients and PUVA phototherapy continued.

All the appropriate cautions for the use of PUVA need to be exercised as outlined in the chapter on psoralen phototherapy in this book. It should be stressed that PUVA needs to be used with great caution in these patients and the amount of UVA exposure gradually and carefully increased. It is possible to worsen the pustular phase of this disease if an excessive phototoxic reaction is obtained. The reader is referred to Chapter 9.

Methotrexate Therapy

If synthetic retinoids are unavailable or cannot be used and if active therapy has to be used, then methotrexate is probably the next drug of choice. Great care has to be taken with the use of this agent in generalized pustular psoriasis. It is critical to avoid overdosing the patients because renal function and clearance of this drug may be significantly reduced in the acute phase of pustular psoriasis. Very low dosages should be used, starting no higher than a 5-mg single weekly dosage either intravenously, intramuscularly, or orally. Full blood counts and biochemistry profiles should be monitored on a regular basis after giving the methotrexate. Full details of methotrexate use are given in Chapter 10.

Hydroxyurea

This has proved a disappointing drug in generalized pustular psoriasis and the author does not use it.

Other Systemic Agents Occasionally Used

SYSTEMIC CORTICOSTEROIDS.—Very rarely, systemic corticosteroids are to be used in life-threatening pustular psoriasis, particularly where the other drugs listed above and the other therapies are either unusable or unobtainable. In addition, when patients have had previous systemic corticosteroids stopped, leading to a generalized pustular flare, these agents should be reintroduced and then slowly tapered. For example, if a patient has had previous extensive topical steroid therapy or previous systemic steroid therapy then 40–60 mg per day of prednisone might be started and then gradually reduced as the patient improves and other treatments, such as retinoids or methotrexate, are begun.

DAPSONE.—Another drug that in the author's experience is of little value in generalized pustular psoriasis is dapsone. One report does suggest that high dosages of dapsone produce a good response, particularly in the infantile form of this disease.[9]

GENERALIZED PUSTULAR PSORIASIS THERAPY: SUMMARY

This is a potentially severe and lethal variant form of psoriasis. Great care has to be taken in its management (Table 15–2).

It is advisable for these patients to be managed by a dermatologist skilled in the management of severe skin problems. Patients ideally should be managed as hospital inpatients with the appropriate care taken in general nursing care as well as consideration of systemic therapy.

If there are any known precipitating factors, for example precipitation of the pustular psoriasis by topical corticosteroid treatments[1, 2] or the occasional precipitation by systemic therapy for other conditions such as lithium

TABLE 15–2.—THERAPY OF GENERALIZED
PUSTULAR PSORIASIS

General Care
    Hospitalize
    Regulate fluid and electrolyte balance
    Bed rest
    Emollients
    If on systemic or topical steroids continue, otherwise
        pustulation will worsen; reduce when more stable
Systemic
    Synthetic retinoids: Treatment of choice
        Etretinate
        Isotretinoin (13-cis-retinoic acid)
        New retinoids
    Methotrexate: With caution!
    Hydroxyurea: Poor response
    Steroids: Only as a last resort!

---

therapy,[5] then these factors should all be reduced or removed from the patient's environment. Great care should be taken with the choice of therapy.

The availability of synthetic retinoids has been a major advance in the management of this condition.

Systemic agents such as methotrexate need to be used with great caution because of the potential for increased toxicity.

REFERENCES

1. Baker H., Ryan T.J.: Generalised pustular psoriasis: A clinical and epidemiological study of 104 cases. *Br. J. Dermatol.* 80:771–793, 1968.
2. Boxley J.D., Dawber R.P.R., Summerly R.: Generalised pustular psoriasis on withdrawal of clobetasol propionate ointment. *Br. Med. J.* 2:225–256, 1975.
3. Hallopeau H.: Sur un quatriene fair d'acrodermatite suppurative continué. *Ann. Dermatol. Syphilol.* 8:1277–1279, 1897.
4. Hebra F.: Schwabgerschaft dem Wochenbette und bei Unterinalkrankheiten der Frauen zu beobachtende Hautkrankheiten. *Wien Med. Wochenschr.* 22:1197–1199, 1872.
5. Lowe N.J., Ridgway H.B.: Generalized pustular psoriasis precipitated by lithium carbonate. *Arch. Dermatol.* 114;1788–1789, 1978.
6. Morison W.L., Parrish J.A., Fitzpatrick T.B.: Oral methoxsalen photochemotherapy of recalcitrant dermatoses of the palms and soles. *Br. J. Dermatol.* 99:297–302, 1978.
7. Orfanos C.E., Landes E., Block P.H.: Trátment du psoriasis postulense par un nouveau retinoid aromative (RO 10 9359). *Ann. Dermatol. Venereol.* 105:807, 1978.
8. Sofen H., Moy R., Lowe N.J.: Isotretinoin for generalised pustular psoriasis. *Lancet* 40, 1984.
9. Staughton R.: Infantile generalized pustular psoriasis responding to Dapsone. *Proc. R. Soc. Med.* 70:286–287, 1977.
10. Takigawa M., Miyachi Y., Uehara M., et al.: Treatment of pustulosis palmaris et plantaris with oral doses of colchicine. *Arch. Dermatol.* 118:458–460, 1982.
11. Thune P.: Treatment of palmo-plantar pustulosis with Tigason. *Dermatologica* 164:67–72, 1982.
12. Wilkinson J.D., Ralfs I.G., Harper J.I., et al.: Topical methoxsalen photochemotherapy in the treatment of palmoplantar pustulosis and psoriasis. *Acta Dermatol. Venereol. (Stockh.)* 59 (Suppl. 89):193–198, 1979.
13. Von Zumbusch L.R.: Psoriasis und pustulosus Exanthem. *Arch. Dermatol. Syphilol.* 99:335–344, 1910.

16 / Exfoliative Psoriasis Therapy

NICHOLAS J. LOWE, M.D., F.R.C.P., F.A.C.P.

EXFOLIATIVE PSORIASIS is the occurrence of total or almost total skin involvement with psoriasis. This usually occurs in a patient who has had previous stable psoriasis, although it can arise as the first manifestation of the disease.

For the differential diagnosis of exfoliative psoriasis the reader is referred to Chapter 1, as well as the articles by Abrahams, et al.[1] and Wilson.[5]

POTENTIAL CAUSES OF EXFOLIATIVE PSORIASIS

As noted above, exfoliative psoriasis usually develops in a patient with previously stable chronic psoriasis. More rarely it is the initial manifestation of the disease. When it arises in previously stable psoriasis some of the causes of that exfoliative state are as follows.

These causes include adverse reactions to various forms of phototherapy resulting in ultraviolet-induced erythema or phototoxic erythema. In some patients, the psoriasis may become exfoliative as a result of a Koebner's response in the ultraviolet damaged skin.

Occasionally coal tars or anthralin may produce skin irritation and subsequent exfoliative psoriasis. This is particularly true if anthralin concentrations are increased too rapidly, leading to an irritant dermatitis. Again the reader is referred to the relevant chapters in this book on those forms of therapy.

Another therapeutic cause of exfoliative psoriasis is the extensive use of potent topical corticosteroids or the use of systemic corticosteroids. In this author's experience, the use of these agents and more particularly the sudden withdrawal of these agents may result in either exfoliative psoriasis or generalized pustular psoriasis. When these agents are used they must be used with due caution and they must be slowly reduced in dosage and frequency to try to lessen the risk of exfoliative psoriasis.

Exfoliative psoriasis also may arise when the patient with psoriasis is treated with a drug for other medical reasons. Examples of drugs which may lead to severe worsening of previously stable psoriasis and in some instances exfoliative psoriasis include antimalarials, gold therapy, lithium, and some beta blockers, although such changes may result from an idiopathic reaction to any drug.

MANAGEMENT OF EXFOLIATIVE PSORIASIS

Exfoliative psoriasis can be a potentially dangerous form of psoriasis, particularly in the elderly patient or in the patient with preexisting heart disease. There are a variety of problems that these patients can develop. Patients with previous heart disease and impaired cardiac function can develop high-output cardiac failure.[2, 4, 5] In addition, a significant thermoregulatory disturbance may occur in cold climates and can produce severe hypothermia, which occasionally can be fatal, particularly in the elderly patient. In extremely hot and humid climates, the reverse is possible and hyperthermia can arise in patients with exfoliative psoriasis.[2, 4]

General Measures

In this author's opinion, patients who have severe exfoliative psoriasis should in general be hospitalized until the severe exfoliation has improved. The reasons for hospitalization are to carefully monitor for the potential onset of cardiovascular, thermoregulatory, fluid, and electrolyte problems.

Specific Measures

Careful attention to fluid and electrolyte balance and adequate maintenance of body temperature are important. The frequent use of emollients is an important measure to try to reduce the transepidermal water loss and help relieve the severe discomfort present in many of these patients.

In many patients it is appropriate to use a medium-to-high-potency topical corticosteroid preparation. Where the patient will tolerate an ointment base, the more occlusive corticosteroid ointments are probably more beneficial. It should be noted, however, that in exfoliative psoriasis there is probably a high percutaneous absorption of the corticosteroid; thus, care has to be taken not to continue these preparations for too long. The ideal is to use the topical corticosteroids twice daily with additional liberal use of emollients for sufficient time to produce a reduction of the exfoliative psoriasis.

An alternative therapy following this initial reduction of severe exfoliative erythroderma is the use of modified Goeckerman regimen. In the author's experience this is often a very satisfactory form of therapy to use following topical corticosteroid therapy in exfoliative psoriasis. Again the reader is referred to the appropriate chapters on emollients, topical corticosteroids and ultraviolet phototherapy.

Another extremely valuable form of treatment for exfoliative psoriasis is synthetic retinoid therapy. The synthetic retinoid etretinate is very effective as a therapy for exfoliative psoriasis.[3] At the present time, etretinate is not approved by the Food and Drug Administration in the United States; it is, however, available in Canada and in Europe. It is available for investigative use at select centers in the United States. It is a much more effective synthetic retinoid for the therapy of this type of psoriasis than is 13-cis-retinoic acid (N.J. Lowe, unpublished data).

Plate 10 shows the difference in response to these two retinoids in a patient with exfoliative psoriasis. This patient, who had exfoliative psoriasis, was treated for four months with oral 13-cis-retinoic acid (dosage 1.5 mg/kg body weight). She failed to respond at all to this therapy. It was then possible to start her on a course of etretinate therapy and within six weeks a dramatic improvement in exfoliative psoriasis occurred, as shown. The reader is referred to Chapter 11 for the details of patient selection and management with these drugs.

Another form of therapy that is often extremely effective in the treatment of exfoliative psoriasis is the use of systemic methotrexate. Again, this is usually administered by the oral route although it may be given intramuscularly or intravenously. The reader is referred to Chapter 10 for the details of methotrexate therapy. Caution needs to be exercised with the use of methotrexate in all patients, but particular caution is needed in patients with more severe forms of psoriasis, particularly exfoliative psoriasis and generalized pustular psoriasis. In exfoliative psoriasis there may be significant prerenal dehydration, a reduced urinary output, and therefore a reduced renal excretion of the methotrexate. Therefore, careful monitoring of the patient is necessary, with frequent complete blood count and platelet count plus blood biochemistry profiles.

PUVA therapy using oral 8-methoxypsoralen is disappointing in the therapy of exfoliative psoriasis. This may be partly because it is not possible to watch for any phototoxic erythema because the patient is totally erythro-dermic. In this author's experience, until severe exfoliative psoriasis has been improved by the measures outlined above, PUVA therapy should not be used.

REFERENCES

1. Abrahams I., McCarthy J.T., Sanders S.L.: One hundred and one cases of exfoliative der-matitis. *Arch. Dermatol.* 87:96–101, 1963.
2. Fox R.H., Shuster S., Williams R., et al.: Cardiovascular, metabolic and thermoregulatory disturbances in patients with erythrodermic skin diseases. *Br. Med. J.* 1:619–622, 1965.
3. Kaplan R.P., Russell D.H., Lowe N.J.: Etretinate therapy for psoriasis. *J. Am. Acad. Dermatol.* 8:95–102, 1983.
4. Shuster S.: Systemic effects of skin disease. *Lancet* 1:907–912, 1967.
5. Wilson H.T.H.: Exfoliative dermatitis: Its etiology and prognosis. *Arch. Dermatol.* 69:577–588, 1954.

17 / Nail Psoriasis Therapy

RONALD L. MOY, M.D.

NICHOLAS J. LOWE, M.D., F.R.C.P., F.A.C.P.

NAILS ARE COMMONLY involved in psoriasis. Although the reported incidence of nail involvement can vary depending on the study, in one series almost 50% of patients had nail involvement.[3] The incidence of nail involvement may depend on the severity of skin involvement, although Pilsbury, et al.[12] state that in their experience nail changes are no more likely in severe cases of psoriasis than in mild ones. Nail changes are said to be more common on the fingers than the toes[15]; however, this may be because toenail involvement is less disturbing to the patient and therefore not mentioned to the physician. Nail involvement can occur as the sole manifestation of psoriasis.[9] Patients with psoriatic arthritis more commonly have psoriatic alterations of the nail than patients with only skin manifestations.[7]

The changes in psoriasis of the nails include pits, discoloration (including "oil spots"), onycholysis, subungual thickening, loss of luster, crumbling, and grooving.

Pits are the most common psoriatic nail defect (Plate 11). The pits are usually less than 1 mm in diameter and quite shallow. Pitting may vary from a few isolated pits on one nail to involvement of all nails. Furrows and depressions can be seen in psoriasis. Onycholysis, or nail detachment from the nail bed, occurs almost as often as pitting (Plate 12). The separation most commonly starts at the edge of the nail and involves only a part of the nail. A yellowish or brown discoloration often occurs around areas of onycholysis, separating the pink normal nail from the white separated area. This yellow color is rarely seen in onycholysis attributed to other causes. These areas of the nail bed when seen through the nail plate resemble oil spots. Subungual hyperkeratosis is a common cause of secondary bacterial and fungal infections in psoriatic nails.[6]

159

HISTOLOGY

The pathologic changes of psoriasis of the nail show many of the same changes found in psoriatic skin. The changes in acute psoriasis of the fingernail include acanthosis, elongation of the rete ridges, severe hyperkeratosis, neutrophils in the epidermis sometimes forming Munro microabscesses, and thinning of the suprapapillary plate.[8] Pits are a result of parakeratosis in the part of the matrix that forms the superficial layer of the nail plate. These areas of parakeratotic horn are weaker than the surrounding normal nail plate and fall off, resulting in a pit. Onycholysis, subungual keratosis, the "oil spots" and discoloration result from nail bed or hyponychium involvement. Parakeratosis, acanthosis, and lack of a granular layer are all seen in the nail bed or hyponychium of these nail changes.[15]

TREATMENT

Wilan, in 1808,[14] stated that the nail changes are part of the psoriatic process and that treatment of the disease itself will give better results than local therapy alone. It is true that psoriasis of the nails often improves spontaneously and may improve as the skin lesions resolve. Therapy with methotrexate, PUVA, ultraviolet-B therapy, and systemic retinoids have all been reported to improve psoriatic nails.[4, 10] Local nail treatment methods are available that can bring improvement in nail psoriasis, although each method has major disadvantages.

High-potency topical steroids applied to the nail matrix under occlusion may be helpful. This therapy must be continued for three months because of the slow growth of the nails. The problem with this method of therapy is that soft-tissue atrophy often occurs before any normal nail growth appears.

Intradermal nail fold injection of triamcinolone acetonide has been shown to produce results in patients with psoriatic nail dystrophy. Triamcinolone acetonide in a concentration of 5 mg/cc is injected into the nail fold just proximal to the diseased matrix. Approximately 0.1 cc is infiltrated in each of three wheels around the matrix. The Dermojet produces less pain than a 30-gauge needle for injection. The steroid injections produce improvement in 80%–90% of patients with nail-matrix changes (other than onycholytic changes) and improvement in 26%–49% of the patients with onycholytic changes.[1, 2, 11] Problems associated with the injections are relapses of the nail dystrophy, the possibility of skin atrophy, and pain at the injection site.

TABLE 17–1.—THE CONTENTS OF 40% UREA PASTE
TO REMOVE HYPERTROPHIC NAILS

INGREDIENT	%	AMOUNT (gm)	
Urea	40	120	200
White beeswax (or soft paraffin)	5	15	25
Anhydrous lanolin	20	60	100
White petrolatum	25	75	125
Silica gel type H	10	30	50
		300	500

Topically applied 1% fluorouracil solution produces apparent decrease of pitting and hypertrophy in patients with psoriatic nail dystrophy. The 1% fluorouracil solution is applied twice daily around the margin of the nail fold. No occlusion is used. Patients with pronounced onycholysis should not be treated with this method because a worsening of the onycholysis has occurred.[5] The response, however, is often disappointing.

Hypertrophic psoriastic nails can be removed by using a urea paste to avulse the nail (Table 17–1). Forty percent urea ointment is applied over the thickened nails after the surrounding paronychial surfaces have been covered with cloth adhesive tape. The patient must keep the nails dry for seven days at which time he or she returns and the nails are removed with a periosteal elevator. A potent topical steroid is applied to the denuded nail bed and proximal nail fold, resulting in approximately a 50% success rate in growing "normal nails."[13]

The treatment of nail psoriasis is largely unsatisfactory. Periungual injections of triamcinolone may a useful treatment but can only be used in patients able to withstand the discomfort of injections. Rapid relapse may occur.

Some patients receiving systemic therapy for psoriasis find they have an improvement of their nail psoriasis. This may occur when patients are treated with PUVA phototherapy, methotrexate, or synthetic retinoids. This response is probably a direct effect on nail psoriasis.

A summary of treatment alternatives for nail psoriasis appears in Table 17–2.

TABLE 17–2.—NAIL PSORIASIS
TREATMENTS

Intradermal nail fold injections of triamcinolone
High potency topical steroids
1% fluorouracil
40% urea ointment
Systemic therapy
  Methotrexate
  PUVA
  Retinoids

REFERENCES

1. Abell E., Samman P.D.: Intradermal triamcinolone treatment of nail dystrophies. *Br. J. Dermatol.* 89:191–197, 1973.
2. Bleeker J.J.: Intralesional triamcinolone acetonide using the Port-O-Jet and needle injections in localized dermatoses. *Br. J. Dermatol.* 91:97–101, 1974.
3. Crawford G.M.: Psoriasis of the nails. *Arch. Dermatol. Syphilol.* 38:583–594, 1938.
4. Dawber R.P.R.: The effect of methotrexate, corticosteroids and azathioprine on fingernail growth in psoriasis. *Br. J. Dermatol.* 83:680–683, 1970.
5. Fredriksson T.: Topically applied fluorouracil in the treatment of psoriatic nails. *Arch. Dermatol.* 110:735–736, 1974.
6. Ganor S.: Chronic paronychia and psoriasis. *Br. J. Dermatol.* 92:685–687, 1975.
7. Krebs A.: Zur Klinils und Therapie der Psoriasis arthropathica. *Dermatologica* 124:249–251, 1962.
8. Lewin K., Dewit S., Ferrington R.A.: Pathology of the fingernail in psoriasis. *Br. J. Dermatol.* 86:555–563, 1972.
9. Moy R.L., Lowe N.J. Psoriatic twenty nail dystrophy. Submitted for publication.
10. Perry H.O., Soderstrom C.W., Schulze R.W.: The Goeckerman treatment of psoriasis. *Arch. Dermatol.* 98:178–182, 1968.
11. Peachy R.D.G., Pye R.J., Harman R.R.M.: The treatment of psoriatic nail dystrophy with intradermal steroid injections. *Br. J. Dermatol.* 95:75–78, 1976.
12. Pilsbury D.M., Shelley W.B., Kligman A.M.: *Dermatology*, ed. 1. Philadelphia, W.B. Saunders Co., 1956.
13. South D.A., Farber E.M.: Urea ointment in the nonsurgical avulsion of nail dystrophies—A reappraisal. *Cutis* 25:609–612, 1980.
14. Wilan R.: *Cutaneous Diseases*, ed. 1. Philadelphia, London, J. Johnson, 1808.
15. Zaias N.: Psoriasis of the nail. A clinical-pathologic study. *Arch. Dermatol.* 99:567–579, 1969.

18 / Psoriatic Arthritis

BRIAN S. ANDREWS, M.D.

PSORIATIC ARTHRITIS is an acute inflammatory arthritis affecting single or multiple joints, with a predilection for those of the hands and the feet. It is associated with cutaneous psoriasis, which in the majority of adults precedes the arthritis. In addition, psoriatic arthritis can be associated with tenosynovitis, periostitis, and inflammation at entheses (insertion sites of tendons and ligaments). Remissions and exacerbations occur in the joint disease, which is usually seronegative (IgM rheumatoid factor negative) without subcutaneous nodules. Classically, psoriatic arthritis involves the distal interphalangeal (DIP) joints.

The association between psoriasis and polyarthritis was first noted by Jean Louis Alibert in the early 19th century. Pierre Bazin, a French dermatologist, coined the term "psoriasis arthritique" in 1860. In 1888 a full clinical description was recorded and in 1904 Menzen reviewed several cases and described the entity in detail. Psoriatic arthritis was not accepted as a specific entity by North Americans until the mid-fifties, for until that time the disease was believed to represent coincidental rheumatoid arthritis in patients with psoriasis. With the discovery of rheumatoid factor in 1940 and then the recognition of the LE-cell phenomenon, psoriatic arthritis was classified as a subgroup of seronegative polyarthritis. Subsequent recognition of familial clustering, the characteristic distribution of joint involvement in patients with psoriasis and the formulation of diagnostic criteria for rheumatoid arthritis led ultimately to the first acceptable classification of psoriatic arthritis in 1976.[13] Today, psoriatic arthritis is recognized as a distinct clinical entity.

EPIDEMIOLOGY

Epidemiologic studies were partially responsible for the acceptance of psoriatic arthritis as a distinct entity. In patients with seropositive polyarthritis, the incidence of psoriatic arthritis is 1.23%, compared with an incidence of psoriasis in the general population of 1.22%. When, however, seronegative polyarthritis is studied, the incidence of psoriasis is 20.2%, markedly increased over the control group. Polyarthritis occurs in approximately 7% of patients with psoriasis. In the general population, rheumatoid arthritis occurs in approximately 3.8%, contrasted with psoriatic arthritis in 0.1%. From these studies it is clear that psoriatic arthritis is associated with the seronegative polyarthritis group and represents a distinct clinical entity.[1, 7, 13]

The inheritance of psoriasis and psoriatic arthritis is generally considered to represent a multifactorial event. A family history of psoriasis or psoriatic arthritis is seen in up to one third of patients. When 310 first- and second-degree relatives of 108 patients with psoriatic arthritis were studied, it was found that psoriasis occurred in 21% of the relatives, seronegative arthritis occurred in 21%, and sacroiliitis with or without spondylitis in 7.4%. However, no increase in erosive polyarthritis was found in the relatives.[8] The HLA-B17 haplotype is significantly increased in patients with psoriasis and, to a lesser extent, in patients with psoriatic arthritis. When HLA-B17 occurs in patients with psoriasis, the presence of HLA-B17 in relatives is associated with a high incidence of psoriasis and earlier onset of the disease. HLA-B13 is also increased in patients with psoriasis alone. Absence of HLA-B12 in patients with psoriasis or psoriatic arthritis lessens the chance of occurrence of these entities in relatives. HLA-B27 is increased in patients with sacroiliitis or with any form of psoriatic spondylitis. A recent Canadian study suggests that no clear association exists between psoriatic arthritis and any of the current serologically defined HLA-DR antigens relative to controls.[3] In summary, the inheritance of psoriasis appears to be multifactorial, with genetic associations linked most strongly to B region alleles.[2, 12, 13]

ETIOLOGY

The etiology of psoriasis and psoriatic arthritis is unknown. Genetic aspects have been covered above. Guttate psoriasis in children may be preceded by streptococcal infections. Trauma to a joint in a patient with psoriasis may predispose to localization of synovitis to the injured joint, but this is not a major contributing factor. Abnormalities in skin capillary loops in patients with psoriasis could bear some relationship to psoriatic arthritis if similar vessel changes were also to occur within synovium. It has been proposed that enhanced reactive hyperemic responses of small phalangeal vessels might also contribute to involvement of DIP joints. Immunologic studies in patients with psoriatic arthritis have failed to demonstrate IgM rheumatoid factor in serum, although IgG anti-immunoglobulins (rheumatoid factors) have been found. Immune complexes have been detected in low levels in serum but these are not believed to be involved in the pathogenesis of synovitis or cutaneous disease. Immunoglobulin and complement may be demonstrated occasionally in dermal capillaries and a moderate impairment in the cutaneous response to dinitrochlorobenzene has been noted. Similarly, these are not regarded as specific findings. T lymphocytes have been detected within synovium, but few detailed immunologic studies have been performed on synovial fluid or synovium. The etiology of psoriatic arthritis thus remains unknown and observations to date add very little to our understanding of immunopathologic events involved in the disease.[2, 12]

PATHOLOGY

The subacute synovitis of psoriatic arthritis is nondiagnostic and is similar to that of rheumatoid arthritis.[2, 10, 12] Proliferation of synovial lining cells and mononuclear cell infiltration of synovium occurs but the synovium is devoid of granulomata and lymphoid follicles. Synovial fibrosis, which is absent in the rheumatoid synovium, has been noted in some patients with psoriatic arthritis. Macroscopically, the synovium is identical to rheumatoid synovium with a mild villous proliferation. The inflammatory process tends initially to preserve articular cartilage. Arthroscopically, the joint cavity appears similar to rheumatoid arthritis. The synovium is infiltrated with mononuclear cells, which are predominantly T lymphocytes. While rheumatoid factor cannot be demonstrated within synovial fluid, small quantities of IgM rheumatoid factor have been found in synovial plasma cells. Thus synovial biopsy in psoriatic arthritis is usually only indicated in monoarticular arthritis to exclude an infectious synovitis such as tuberculosis or specific pathology such as pigmented villonodular synovitis.

CLINICAL PRESENTATION

Psoriatic arthritis can occur in either adults or children. In adults with psoriatic arthritis, 84% have psoriasis that precedes the arthritis, occasionally by 20 years. In 10%, skin and joint disease may develop simultaneously, usually with involvement of DIP joints and adjacent nails. In the remaining 6%, a seronegative polyarthritis precedes skin involvement. However, in this group, while the distribution of the arthritis and a family history may suggest psoriatic arthritis, this diagnosis can only be made retrospectively.[7, 13] In childhood disease, the arthritis precedes the onset of psoriasis in up to 52% of patients and skin involvement is more likely to coincide with the onset of arthritis.[4, 11] The polyarthritis of psoriasis is a typical inflammatory arthritis and is characterized by pain in the joint, particularly with motion, morning stiffness, and gelling after rest. On examination, the joints are swollen, tender, and warm, with a reduced range of motion. The activity of the inflammatory process is paralleled by the duration of morning stiffness (i.e., the longer the stiffness persists, the more active the inflammation) and the severity of gelling. Constitutional symptoms, such as fever, fatigue, and weight loss, which are common in patients with rheumatoid arthritis, are uncommon in psoriatic arthritis, although occasional malaise is noted. Importantly, the short- and long-term disability produced by psoriatic arthritis is much less than that seen in rheumatoid arthritis.

In adults, the mean age of onset of psoriasis is 29 years in males and 26 in females, with the onset of the arthritis occurring between 30 and 55 years, similar to rheumatoid arthritis. The sex incidence of psoriatic arthritis varies markedly between studies, but a generally quoted figure would be a female:male ratio of 1.04:1, contrasting with the definite female predominance of 3:1 in rheumatoid arthritis. In children, the mean age of onset for psoriatic arthritis is 9–10 years with a female:male ratio of 2.8:1, similar to that seen in rheumatoid arthritis.

Onset of psoriatic arthritis is usually subacute, although occasionally a "gout-like" acute monoarticular arthritis can occur. In the latter, a crystal-induced synovitis must be excluded by joint aspiration and examination of the fluid under a polarizing microscope. Hyperuricemia may occur in patients with severe generalized psoriasis, particularly those treated with cytotoxic drugs and in a predisposed individual the hyperuricemia may precipitate an acute attack of gout.

CLINICAL TYPES OF PSORIATIC ARTHRITIS

In adults, five distinct clinical subsets of psoriatic arthritis are recognized.[2, 7, 8, 12, 13]

Type 1: asymmetric oligoarthritis.—This represents the most common form of arthritis in psoriasis and accounts for 70% of psoriatic arthritis

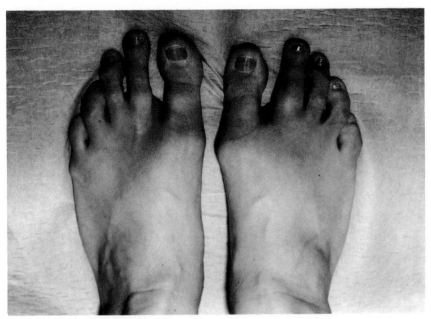

Fig 18–1.—Sausage-shaped swelling of the right second toe in a patient with psoriasis involving the scalp and extensor surfaces.

cases. Typically, two or three joints are involved, usually confined to toes or fingers with involvement in the following descending order: distal interphalangeal (DIP), proximal interphalangeal (PIP), metatarsophalangeal (MTP), and metacarpophalangeal (MCP). However, the oligoarthritis may also involve knees, elbows, wrists, and ankles asymmetrically. This form may be associated with a "sausage digit" (Fig 18–1), representing a combination of DIP and PIP synovitis, flexor tendon tenosynovitis, and soft tissue inflammation with or without periostitis. While "sausage digits" are characteristic of psoriatic arthritis, they are also seen in patients with Reiter's syndrome.

TYPE 2: SYMMETRIC POLYARTHRITIS.—This is clinically very similar to rheumatoid arthritis and occurs in up to 15% of patients with psoriatic arthritis. It is believed to represent a subtype of psoriatic arthritis, rather than rheumatoid arthritis occurring in a patient with psoriasis. The arthritis is frequently nonerosive, has a female predominance, and may be associated with varying low rheumatoid factor titers and an elevated erythrocyte sedimentation rate (ESR).

TYPE 3: CLASSIC PSORIATIC ARTHRITIS.—This arthritis predominantly involves the DIP joints and is frequently associated with severe psoriatic involvement of the nails. This type occurs in from 5%–10% of patients with psoriatic arthritis and has a male predominance.

TYPE 4: DEFORMING POLYARTHRITIS.—This form is severe, produces severe erosive disease, and occurs in 5% of patients with psoriatic arthritis. It is associated with "sausage digits" and marked DIP involvement (Fig 18–2). Whittling of the head of the middle phalanx (pencil) and erosion and splaying of the base (cupping) of the distal phalanx produce the classic "pencil-in-cup" deformity. Uncommonly, this form of arthritis may progress to produce a severe destructive form termed *arthritis mutilans.*

TYPE 5: SPONDYLITIS WITH OR WITHOUT SACROILIITIS.—This occurs in approximately 5% of patients with psoriatic arthritis and has a male predominance. In my experience, however, clinical evidence of spondylitis and/or sacroiliitis can occur in conjunction with other subgroups of psoriatic arthritis. Spondylitis may occur without radiologic evidence of sacroiliitis, which frequently tends to be asymmetric, or may appear radiologically

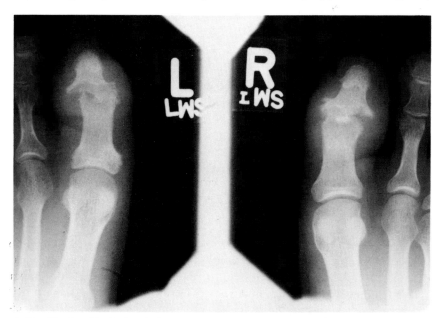

Fig 18–2.—Marked soft tissue swelling and erosive changes affecting the interphalangeal joints of the great toes bilaterally. The erosions, splaying of the base of the distal phalanx, loss of joint space, and destruction of the head of the proximal phalanx are typical of psoriatic arthritis.

without the classical symptoms of morning stiffness in the lower back. Thus, there can be poor correlation between symptoms and radiological signs of sacroiliitis.

Vertebral involvement differs from that seen in ankylosing spondylitis. Vertebrae are affected asymmetrically and the atlantoaxial joint may be involved with erosion of the odontoid and subluxation. There may be unusual radiologic features such as nonmarginal, asymmetric syndesmophytes (characteristic), paravertebral ossification, and less commonly, vertebral fusion with disk calcification.

JUVENILE PSORIATIC ARTHRITIS

The mean age of onset is 9–10 years with a female predominance. As in adults, the disease is usually mild, although occasionally it may be severe and destructive, progressing into adulthood. In 50% of children, the arthritis is monoarticular and DIP involvement occurs in a similar percentage. Tenosynovitis is present in 30%. Nail involvement is present in 71%, with pitting the most common, but least specific finding. In 47%, disordered bone growth with resultant shortening may result from involvement of the unfused epiphyseal growth plate by the inflammatory process. Sacroiliitis occurs in 28% and is usually associated with HLA-B27 positivity. While the presence of HLA-B8 may be a marker of more severe disease, HLA-B17 is usually associated with a mild form of psoriatic arthritis. There is a higher frequency than in adults of simultaneous onset of psoriasis and arthritis, with arthritis preceeding psoriasis in 52%.[4, 11]

SKIN INVOLVEMENT

Arthritis is not generally considered to correlate strongly with any particular type of psoriasis or the severity of the skin disease. However, in one study arthritis was noted more frequently in patients with severe skin disease, while in another, pustular psoriasis was associated with more severe psoriatic arthritis. In patients presenting with an undefined seronegative polyarthritis, it is *extremely* important to look for psoriasis in hidden sites such as the scalp, where psoriasis is frequently mistaken for dandruff, the perineum, the natal cleft, and the umbilicus. A diagnosis of psoriatic arthritis may be missed due to an inadequate physical examination.

NAIL INVOLVEMENT

Involvement of DIP joints correlates moderately well with psoriasis in adjacent nails, although this is not an invariable association. Nails are involved in 80% of patients with psoriatic arthritis, but only in 20% of patients with uncomplicated psoriasis. Severe deforming arthritis of the hands and feet is associated frequently with extensive nail involvement. Three features of nail involvement that should be noted are onycholysis (the most specific), transverse ridging, and uniform nail pitting (the least specific). A direct correlation exists between the number of pits and the diagnostic significance. When skin and joint disease begin simultaneously, nail involvement is frequently present at the onset. Fungal infection of the nails is the main consideration in the differential diagnosis in a patient with a seronegative polyarthritis.

EXTRA-ARTICULAR FEATURES

These are much less frequently observed in patients with psoriatic arthritis than in patients with rheumatoid arthritis. In psoriatic arthritis, there is a predilection for synovitis affecting flexor tendon sheaths with sparing of the extensor tendon sheath; both are commonly involved in rheumatoid arthritis. Subcutaneous nodules are rare in patients with psoriatic arthritis. If nodules are present in a patient who has psoriasis and arthritis, particularly if the rheumatoid factor titer is positive, they suggest the coincidental occurrence of psoriasis and rheumatoid arthritis.

Ocular involvement may occur in 30% of patients with psoriatic arthritis, including conjunctivitis in 20% and acute anterior uveitis in 7%. In patients with uveitis, 43% have sacroiliitis and 40% are HLA-B27 positive. Scleritis and keratoconjunctivitis sicca are rare.[5] Inflammation of the aortic valve root, which may lead to insufficiency, has been described in six patients with psoriatic arthritis, and is similar to that seen more frequently in ankylosing spondylitis and Reiter's syndrome.[10]

LABORATORY DATA

No specific diagnostic tests are available for psoriatic arthritis. The diagnosis of the disease is made on the basis of clinical and radiologic criteria in a patient with psoriasis. IgM RF in serum is usually absent, although low rheumatoid factor titer positivity may be seen intermittently in 16% of patients, particularly those with symmetric polyarthritis. In 33% of patients, however, IgG antiglobulins have been detected in serum. When IgM rheumatoid factor positivity is studied in a group of patients with psoriatic arthritis and a similar comparison undertaken in an age- and sex-matched normal population, rheumatoid factor positivity generally is found to be comparable in both groups. The ESR may be elevated in patients with active psoriatic joint disease but it is uncommon for the ESR (Westergren method) to exceed 100 mm/hour. Severe skin and joint disease may be associated with a mild normochromic normocytic anemia and leukocytosis. Acute phase reactants, such as α-2 macroglobulin, may be increased. Antinuclear antibody titers in psoriatic arthritis do not differ from those of age- and sex-matched control populations. In 10%–20% of patients with generalized skin disease, the serum uric acid may be increased and on occasions predispose to acute gouty arthritis.

Low levels of circulating immune complexes have been detected in 56% of patients with psoriatic arthritis, but levels do not appear to parallel disease activity. The associations of psoriatic arthritis with HLA-B17, HLA-B13, HLA-B27 and HLA-B12 were described earlier. Serum IgA levels are increased in two thirds of patients with psoriatic arthritis and in one third with psoriasis. Levels of IgM tend to increase with severe disease, but IgG levels are usually not elevated.

Synovial fluid is inflammatory, with cell counts ranging from 5,000 to 15,000/mm^3 and with greater than 50% of the cells polymorphonuclear leukocytes. Within the synovium, the infiltrate consists predominantly of T lymphocytes. Synovial fluid complement levels are either normal or increased and glucose levels are normal.

RADIOLOGIC FEATURES

These have helped distinguish psoriatic arthritis from other causes of polyarthritis. In general, the common subtypes of psoriatic arthritis, such as asymmetric oligoarthritis and symmetric polyarthritis, tend to result in only mild erosive disease. Early bony erosions occur at the cartilaginous edge and, initially, cartilage is preserved with maintenance of a normal joint space. Juxtaarticular osteopenia, which is the hallmark of rheumatoid arthritis, is minimal in psoriatic arthritis. Asymmetric erosive changes in small joints of the hands and feet are typical of psoriatic arthritis and have a predilection in decreasing order for DIP, PIP, MTP and MCP joints. Erosive disease frequently occurs in patients with either DIP involvement or progressive deforming arthritis and may lead to subluxation and less commonly bony ankylosis of the joint. Erosion of the tuft of the distal phalanx, and even metatarsals, can progress to complete dissolution of the bone. While this form of acro-osteolysis is not diagnostic, it is very suggestive of psoriatic arthritis. The "pencil in cup" deformity seen in hands and feet of patients with severe joint disease usually affects the DIP joints (see Fig 18–2) but may also involve PIP joints.

Involvement of the axial skeleton in psoriatic arthritis is common and not mutually exclusive of peripheral joint involvement. Sacroiliitis can be demonstrated radiologically in 20% of patients with spinal involvement, tends to be asymmetric initially (similar to Reiter's syndrome) and need not parallel clinical involvement. Nonmarginal syndesmophytes are most common in the lumbar spine but may also involve isolated thoracic and cervical vertebrae. These bony projections are asymmetric (also typical of Reiter's syndrome) and originate from the anterior or lateral aspects of the vertebral body. They differ from the marginal syndesmophytes seen in ankylosing spondylitis and colitic spondylitis. Another characteristic feature of psoriatic spondylitis is involvement of the atlantoaxial joint, which may result in erosion of the odontoid and subluxation of C1 on C2. This change is similar to that seen more frequently in rheumatoid arthritis. Fusion of thoracic vertebrae and paravertebral ossification are uncommon in psoriatic arthritis and the "bamboo spine" of ankylosing spondylitis is rarely seen. With all forms of vertebral and sacroiliac involvement in psoriatic arthritis, there is a high association of HLA-B27 positivity.[2, 6, 12]

DIFFERENTIAL DIAGNOSIS

REITER'S SYNDROME.—This syndrome, most frequently diagnosed in males but also occurring in females, follows venereal or gastrointestinal infection. It represents a form of "reactive arthritis" and consists of a clinical triad of urethritis, conjunctivitis, and arthritis. Synovitis of the knee joint, usually with a large effusion, followed by involvement of the ankle, and a "sausage digit," most frequently in a toe, are the common articular manifestations in Reiter's syndrome. The arthritis is either monoarticular or asymmetric pauciarticular. Painless mouth ulcers do not occur in psoriasis and circinate balanitis is more suggestive of Reiter's syndrome.

ACUTE HEBERDEN'S NODE(S).—This represents an asymmetric acute inflammatory process involving the DIP joint(s) of the fingers and occasionally may be mistaken for psoriatic arthritis. When present, there is usually clinical and radiologic evidence of cartilaginous or bony proliferation (osteophytes) at the base of the distal phalanx and frequently associated with a past or family history of osteoarthritis. In osteoarthritis, the PIP and first carpometacarpal joints are also frequently involved. The less common, erosive osteoarthritis must also be considered.

ACUTE GOUTY ARTHRITIS.—This may occur in psoriatic arthritis and may result from hyperuricemia seen with exfoliative psoriasis, particularly when treated with cytotoxic agents. The initial attack of gout usually begins in the lower limbs, particularly distal to the knee joint. Acute monoarticular arthritis developing in toes, MTPs, or ankle joints in a patient with psoriasis initially should be regarded as gout, irrespective of the serum uric acid level. The involved joint should be aspirated and the synovial fluid examined under polarizing microscopy to identify the needle-like, negatively birefringent urate crystals characteristic of gout. If synovial fluid cannot be obtained, any blood in the needle resulting from the aspiration also should be examined for crystals. Absence of crystals in an acutely inflamed joint suggests that gout is not the diagnosis.

CELLULITIS OR SEPTIC ARTHRITIS.—Occasionally the onset of psoriatic arthritis with soft tissue and tendon sheath inflammation may be misdiagnosed as cellulitis. The latter is usually associated with an abrasion in the skin, fever, and lymphangitis. If infection is suspected, the soft tissue should be aspirated, the aspirate cultured and the patient commenced on the appropriate antibiotic(s). A suspected septic joint must be aspirated, a Gram stain and white cell count determined, and the fluid cultured. Antibiotics should be given until the results of the culture are obtained. Note that if the joint can be readily moved without pain, it is less likely to be involved by gout or a septic process.

TRAUMATIC ARTHRITIS.—This may occur in a patient with psoriasis, with the knee the most commonly involved joint. If the joint remains tender and swollen, particularly after minimal trauma, psoriatic arthritis should be considered. Synovial fluid should be removed and if a doubt still persists, arthrography and/or arthroscopy with biopsy should be undertaken.

RHEUMATOID ARTHRITIS.—As both psoriasis and rheumatoid arthritis occur frequently in the population and one is not mutually exclusive of the other, rheumatoid arthritis may occur in a patient with psoriasis. The presence of symmetric polyarthritis associated with subcutaneous nodules and a positive rheumatoid factor in a patient with psoriasis suggests rheumatoid arthritis. As rheumatoid arthritis is common and as a monoarticular presentation occurs in 25% of patients with rheumatoid arthritis, monoarticular arthritis in a patient with psoriasis and rheumatoid factor positivity in serum and synovial fluid may also represent early onset of rheumatoid arthritis in a patient with psoriasis.

MANAGEMENT

Improvement in psoriatic skin disease is frequently associated with remission of the arthritis. However, both skin and joint disease should be managed individually.

The patient with extensive psoriasis is usually extremely distressed. Therefore, the development of arthritis may be emotionally devastating. Thus, the management of skin and joint disease and the psyche is extremely important. Further, with any chronic disease, a chronic pain syndrome such as the fibromyalgic syndrome (fibrositis) may develop and one should be aware of this defined clinical entity and its management.

PSORIATIC ARTHRITIS

General Considerations

For any patient with arthritis, there are important general principles of management. With inflammatory joint disease associated with prolonged morning stiffness, gelling, pain, and fatigue, the patient and joints require rest. The hands, which are frequently involved, may require splinting. These may be activity splints, which help patients perform their normal daily functions, or rest splints, which are applied during periods when the joints are not in use in an attempt to maintain a position of function, protect the joint, and help lessen inflammation. Paraffin soaks of the hands produce symptomatic relief and do not appear to adversely affect local skin disease. With active synovitis of joints or flexor tendons, it is important that range of motion exercises of involved joints be undertaken several times each day to maintain normal function and limit development of contractures. In spite of aggressive occupational and physical therapy, patients with a destructive arthropathy affecting hands and feet may still develop subluxation of joints, contractures, and even bony ankylosis unless remittive therapy is instituted. Patient education and reassurance are extremely important, particularly as the majority of patients with psoriatic arthritis will have a relatively mild, nonerosive arthritis. In many patients, psoriatic arthritis may remain undiagnosed, particularly if the skin disease represents the more dominant inflammatory process.

Joint Aspiration

This may be required to exclude a septic process or crystal-induced synovitis. Joints can be aspirated relatively safely through psoriatic skin lesions provided the skin is not infected and an aseptic technique is employed. However aspiration through normal skin is preferable. Although there are several case reports of patients developing septic arthritis following aspiration, the benefits of aspiration will far outweigh the risks if appropriate precautions are undertaken.

Nonsteroidal Anti-inflammatory Drugs (NSAIDs)

These drugs afford symptomatic relief of the joint disease by producing analgesia and reducing inflammation. They will not produce a remission and, if given to a patient with progressive erosive deforming disease, will not affect the ultimate outcome. With any of the NSAIDs there is no way to predict which drug will be effective in a given patient or which drug will produce side effects. The NSAIDs that I would use for the typical adult patient, in order of preference, are:

INDOMETHACIN (INDOCIN).—A usual dose is 50–150 mg/day given three or four times daily with food or antacids. The common side effects with this drug are gastrointestinal, including nausea, pain, diarrhea, or gastric bleeding; central nervous system disturbances, particularly in the elderly; and sodium and fluid retention. The latter may be of concern in patients with hypertension and congestive heart failure. Indocin SR (75 mg), a sustained release form, may be taken orally once or twice daily to optimize compliance. Indomethacin suppositories (50 mg) recently have become available and are particularly useful when used at night for relieving nocturnal pain and morning stiffness.

SULINDAC (CLINORIL).—This drug is my second choice if indomethacin is not effective or produces significant side effects. The usual dosage is 200 mg twice daily with meals.

TOLMETIN SODIUM (TOLECTIN).—Tolectin 200 mg or 400 mg is taken four times a day with meals or antacids, up to a maximum dose of 2 gm/day if tolerated. Gastrointestinal intolerance and fluid retention also occur with Tolectin.

NAPROXEN SODIUM (NAPROSYN, ANAPROX).—The usual dosage employed is 250–500 mg twice daily with meals.

ASPIRIN.—This can be employed in anti-inflammatory doses up to 3.6 gm/day, although generally it is less effective in psoriatic arthritis than it is in rheumatoid arthritis. In individual patients, however, aspirin can be extremely effective and if a good response is obtained, aspirin should be maintained in a full anti-inflammatory dose to produce an optimal plasma salicylate level between 15–25 mg/dl.

Few data are currently available with drugs such as piroxicam (Feldene) 20 mg/daily, but this appears to be an effective therapy.

Remittive Agents

These drugs are required in patients developing progressive, erosive psoriatic arthritis or who have active polyarthritis poorly controlled with NSAIDs. If erosions develop, a remittive agent should be commenced early to arrest the joint destruction.[2, 12]

METHOTREXATE.—This drug is frequently used by dermatologists for severe psoriasis and is the first remittive agent I would employ. Commonly, patients with severe psoriasis are referred to a rheumatologist for management of arthritis and by mutual agreement methotrexate is the agent employed for treating both skin and joint diseases. General rules followed for the use of methotrexate include:

1. It should not be used in patients with established liver disease, e.g., chronic active hepatitis or cirrhosis, or if the patient is an alcoholic.

2. It can be administered either as a single weekly dose or three doses at 12 hourly intervals once weekly to limit the risk of hepatic fibrosis. I begin with a 5–7.5 mg dose and increase this to between 15–25 mg as a single weekly dose. When methotrexate is used in this manner the patient can be followed carefully and laboratory parameters (CBC, liver function tests) monitored carefully.

3. The role of liver biopsy is controversial. Prior to initiation of methotrexate, a liver biopsy can be performed, although this is not uniform clini-

cal practice. Most would agree that liver biopsies are required if liver function tests remain persistently elevated, while others perform an annual liver biopsy on patients on long-term methotrexate or after a total dose of 2.5 gm has been administered. Common side effects seen with these doses include hepatitis which can result in hepatic fibrosis, leukopenia, thrombocytopenia, and mucosal ulceration.

For further information, the reader is referred to Chapter 10.

GOLD.—Aurothioglucose (Solganal) is given in the same way as for rheumatoid arthritis, with initial weekly intramuscular test doses of 10 mg and 25 mg followed by a regular maintenance intramuscular dose of 50 mg weekly. Skin reactions can occur in 30% of patients, but generally these are mild. Routine CBC and urinalysis are performed weekly prior to the gold injection to insure that the white cell count exceeds 4,000/cu mm, the platelet count exceeds 100,000/cu mm and that significant proteinuria (i.e., +1 or more) is not present. Should significant proteinuria develop, a 24-hour urinary protein level should be performed before further gold is given.

ANTIMALARIALS, E.G., HYDROXYCHLOROQUINE SULFATE (PLAQUENIL).—Until recently antimalarials had been avoided in psoriasis because of the fear of exacerbating the skin disease. Several case reports have documented this complication, but in larger studies it appears that the effects of antimalarials on the skin disease are minimal. As this fear still persists and as a remission of the psoriatic arthritis may only occur in less than two thirds of patients on antimalarials, these drugs are still generally not used.

MERCAPTOPURINE (PURINETHOL) OR AZATHIOPRINE (IMURAN).—There is little conclusive data to support the use of these drugs, although they are effective in isolated patients with progressive Reiter's syndrome. Azathioprine may be indicated in severe progressive erosive psoriatic arthritis if methotrexate and gold are either ineffective or produce undue side effects.

Corticosteroids

Systemic corticosteroids should be avoided in the management of psoriatic arthritis. While steroids may be effective in alleviating symptoms, they are *not* remittive agents and high doses are usually required to produce significant symptomatic relief of the polyarthritis. Local steroids can be extremely effective when injected into inflamed joints or tendon sheaths. A significant local effect can be observed within 2–3 days and allows maintenance of range of movement and limitation of flexor tendon contractures. Further, local injections into the nail bed for psoriatic involvement may also lessen the inflammatory process in the adjacent DIP joint.

Surgery

Indications for surgery in psoriatic arthritis are similar to those in rheumatoid arthritis. From a practical point of view, surgery is most commonly required for fingers and toes. In the fingers, surgery includes joint replacement with prosthestic silastic implants or joint fusion; in the toes, resection of metatarsal heads may be indicated. Incisions through psoriatic plaques do not appear to be associated with a higher incidence of postoperative joint infection than in patients with rheumatoid arthritis.

SUMMARY

Psoriatic arthritis is a relatively common inflammatory polyarthritis. It is usually mild to moderate in severity and is infrequently associated with severe erosive joint disease. If erosive disease develops, it should be treated early and aggressively with remittive agents to halt progression of the inflammatory process. Optimal management of psoriatic arthritis can be achieved by a close working relationship between internist, dermatologist, and rheumatologist.

REFERENCES

1. Baker H.: Epidemiological aspects of psoriasis and arthritis. *Br. J. Dermatol.* 78:249–261, 1966.
2. Bennett R.M.: Psoriatic arthritis, in McCarty D.J. (ed.): *Arthritis*, ed. 9. Philadelphia, Lea & Febiger, 1979, pp. 642–655.
3. Gladman D., Anhorn K.B., Mervert H., et al.: HLA antigens in psoriatic arthritis—lack of association with DR antigens. Scientific Abstracts. 48th Annual Meeting American Rheumatism Association S85:D57, 1984.
4. Lambert J.R., Ansell B.M., Stephenson E., et al.: Psoriatic arthritis in childhood. *Clin. Rheum. Dis.* 2:339–352, 1976.
5. Lambert J.R., Wright V.: Eye inflammation in psoriatic arthritis. *Ann. Rheum. Dis.* 35:354–356, 1976.
6. Lambert J.R., Wright V.: Psoriatic spondylitis: A clinical and radiological description of the spine in psoriatic arthritis. *Quart. J. Med.* 46:411–425, 1977.
7. Leczinsky C.G.: The incidence of arthropathy in a ten year series of psoriasis cases. *Acta Dermatol. Venereol.* 28:483–487, 1948.

8. Moll J.M.H., Wright V.: Familial occurrence of psoriatic arthritis. *Ann. Rheum. Dis.* 32:181–201, 1973.
9. Reed W.B., Becker S.W., Rohde R., et al.: Psoriasis and arthritis. Clinicopathologic study. *Arch. Dermatol.* 83:541–548, 1961.
10. Sherman M.: Psoriatic arthritis. Observation on the clinical, roentgenographic and pathological changes. *J. Bone Joint Surg.* 34A:831–852, 1952.
11. Sills E.M.: Psoriatic arthritis in childhood. *Johns Hopkins Med. J.* 146:49–53, 1980.
12. Wright V.: Psoriatic arthritis, in Kelley W.N., et al. (eds.): *Textbook of Rheumatology,* ed. 1. Philadelphia, W.B. Saunders Co., 1981, pp. 1047–1062.
13. Wright V., Moll J.M.H.: *Seronegative Polyarthritis.* Amsterdam, North-Holland, 1976.

19 / Psoriasis Treatment: Useful Information and Instructions for Patients

NICHOLAS LOWE, M.D., F.R.C.P., F.A.C.P.

THE AUTHOR uses this section as a handout for psoriasis patients in the hope it provides them with useful information.

To the psoriasis patient: The purpose of this handout is to provide the patient an overview of psoriasis treatment currently available. Many patients can be treated on an outpatient basis by topical medications alone; a small percent of patients will require programs provided by a day-care center or inpatient hospital setting.

Virtually all patients with psoriasis can be improved to a state where they can lead normal lives; however, different treatments are necessary for different patients. You may have had psoriasis for a long time and know a lot about it, and you may have had many of the treatments to be outlined; or this may be the first time that you have been told that this is your problem. In this case, even if you have only mild psoriasis, it is not the purpose of this information to scare or depress you. It is the purpose to inform you about the condition so that you can better understand your situation.

Psoriasis is a chronic scaling disease with skin redness or inflammation. It can be there all the time but it may also go away or be improved for long periods.

The plan in psoriasis treatment is to improve your psoriasis to a degree that is physically and socially acceptable to you.

Different treatment programs are available. It is very important that all family members (parents, spouses, and close friends) understand the treatment program so they may provide support. You should read all the material given to you. Individual questions can be answered during visits as they arise. It often helps to bring family or close friends with you to your visits with your physician.

TREATMENT

What Makes Psoriasis Worse

1. TRAUMA AND IRRITATION TO YOUR SKIN.—One of the most important points is that *injury to* or *irritation of* the skin may result in psoriasis. Rubbing, scratching, or scrubbing off scales, rubbing, brushing or picking at the scalp, sunburn, and local infection—all can produce psoriasis. You should not scratch or rub your skin.

The development of psoriasis after injury has been reported after surgical or accidental scars, burns, dermatitis (e.g., contact dermatitis, like poison ivy), bites, drug reaction, prickly heat, sun rashes, seborrheic dermatitis, pityriasis rosea, ringworm (fungus), thumb sucking, vaccination, herpes, shingles, and other infections of the skin.

2. SUN EXPOSURE.—*Sunlight in moderation usually helps psoriasis* but *sunburn* may cause psoriasis *to flare up.* A small percent (10%) of people may be made worse by any amount of sun. You should, therefore, use a sunscreen based on your skin type. The newer swim suits that allow sunburning should be used with sunscreens.

3. INFECTIONS.—Primarily some throat and upper respiratory infections may flare psoriasis and *should be promptly treated by your physician.* Guttate (drop-like spots) psoriasis particularly occurs in children and adolescents after strep throat activity.

4. TOPICAL STEROIDS OR CORTISONES.—Topical cortisones are very easy to use; *however if other medications are not added then the psoriasis quickly returns.* Topical cortisone should not be used on areas in which the psoriasis is cleared (when the skin is flat, even though it may be still a little brown). Misuse of topical cortisone—putting strong steroid (e.g., Diprolene, Lidex, Halog, Synalar, Valisone) on skin too often and for too long—can lead to change in skin color, pimples, stretch marks, thinning of the skin and easy bruising. Face and skin creases or folds (body folds) are special danger areas for these drugs.

5. OTHER DRUGS.—Some drugs given for other diseases may make psoriasis worse. These may affect some but not all patients. Check with your dermatologist.

Some *drugs* that may *worsen* your *psoriasis:*
Lithium
Gold
Indomethacin
Beta blockers, such as Inderal
Antimalarials

6. STRESS AND ANXIETY.—Some patients find that stress makes their psoriasis worse. If this seems to occur try to find ways of stress control or reduction, such as relaxation programs. If this remains a problem then psychological counseling may be helpful.

7. DIET.—No consistent dietary link with psoriasis has been found; however, certain guidelines may be important.
1. A healthy mixed diet is important for general health.
2. Psoriasis patients may find their problem worse if they are overweight. Correct weight is important also for good health.
3. It is possible that for theoretical reasons a diet rich in fish or in certain essential fatty acids may improve psoriasis. However, no controlled investigations have as yet been conducted. For example, some years ago a diet rich in white turkey meat was found not to be helpful as had been previously suggested in uncontrolled studies.

Salicylic Acid

This agent works by breaking down and peeling off excess scale in the psoriatic areas.

Tar

It is known that application of coal tar improves psoriasis lesions. It probably works by slowing the rate of cell growth in the skin. These medications often work better when combined with cautious ultraviolet therapy.

The purified tars have made using tar much easier; they are much better suited to an outpatient program than crude tars.

Estar, Psorigel, T-Derm Oil, P and S Plus are purified tars in cosmetic bases.

Lubricant Emollients and Preparations

Some examples of lubrication or emollient preparations are: Nivea Cream, Eucerin Cream, Aquaphor Cream, Keri Lotion, and Lubriderm. These are aimed at lubricating the skin. They can be used over cortisone cream or ointment and can be used on the skin in between applications of topical medication. They can be used on any dry areas, or on areas where the psoriasis is no longer present.

Some (e.g., Vaseline, white petrolatum) are useful before ultraviolet therapy because they increase the effectiveness of the ultraviolet on psoriasis.

Anthralin

This is an old topical medication available in ointment, cream, stick or paste forms. It has recently been reinvestigated and newer, more convenient treatment schedules described. It is a synthetic substance made from anthracene, a coal tar derivative, and has been used in the treatment of psoriasis since the 19th century.

The disadvantages of anthralin are that it is messy and may stain clothes, skin, and hair, as well as irritate the skin. However, if directions for its use are followed, this can be minimized.

The use of anthralin creams or ointments applied to the skin for short time periods has become known as *short-contact anthralin*. This has the advantage of producing fewer problems of staining of skin and clothes, and skin irritation may be less with this method.

Plastic Occlusion of Skin

The technique of occlusion (wrapping) uses thin plastic or vinyl to increase the penetration of the topical medication into the psoriatic skin. It is usually used with topical cortisones and should be used only under the guidance of a dermatologist. It increases dramatically the skin absorption of topical cortisones, thereby sometimes improving effectiveness; however, potential side effects also increase.

Antihistamines, Sedatives

In cases where itching is severe at night, an antihistamine taken by mouth, such as Atarax, Vistaril, or Benadryl, or a sedative such as Valium may be given for nighttime.

SPECIAL AREAS

Scalp

The scalp is a common site of psoriasis. Psoriasis may remain confined to the scalp or may appear on other areas of the body. Scalp psoriasis often responds slowly and poorly. It may return immediately after treatment is stopped, or it may remain in remission for varying times. It can get worse or better on its own. It often needs special types of treatment that your dermatologist will advise. Some examples are:

1. Cortisone lotion or solution—examples: Diprosone, Halog, Lidex, Valisone. These work in the same way as other topical cortisones, by decreasing cell (skin) growth and inflammation. See previous section for discussion of topical cortisone.

2. Scalp gels, oils, lotions, creams, ointments. These help to either remove psoriasis scales and/or slow down the growth of the psoriasis. They usually contain tars and salicylic acid, often in combination.

3. Shampoos. These are regarded as important medications in scalp treatment. Tar-containing shampoos are probably the best (Pentrax, Sebutone, T-Gel, Vanseb T).

4. Maintenance treatment. Use your tar shampoos at least twice a week even if clear to try to maintain clearance of your scalp psoriasis.

Ears

In some patients, psoriasis of the ear canal can be very stubborn and may impair hearing. Local treatments of the ear canal may clear the psoriasis. Care must be taken not to irritate the ear drum and ear canal. The dermatologist may advise you to see an ear specialist.

Nails

Psoriasis may affect the nails in several ways. It may appear as pits in the nails. It may lift the nails away from the nail bed (onycholysis), and may lead to a collection of material underneath the nail. The nails may become greatly thickened.

Nail psoriasis is very difficult to treat. An important aim for the psoriasis patient is to reduce nail damage to a minimum. Avoidance of damage often helps the nails to improve.

Sometimes nails will improve when internal drugs are taken. Topical medication is usually not effective in nail psoriasis. PUVA is occasionally helpful for nail psoriasis. If nails become greatly thickened, special pastes containing high concentrations of urea may be prescribed by the dermatologist to remove the nails.

FOR PATIENTS WITH MORE SEVERE PSORIASIS: TREATMENT CENTER OR HOSPITAL PROGRAMS

Phototherapy (Tar and Ultraviolet-B Light): The Goeckerman Program

The Goeckerman program, as it is used today to clear psoriasis, is one of the most effective treatment programs, has few side effects, and in a treatment center setting is cost effective. It is not a cure but an excellent way of improving your psoriasis. In the early 1920s the Goeckerman program was described by Dr. W. H. Goeckerman. He observed that this program not only cleared psoriasis, but that it often produced long remissions of the disease. His original method has been modified, but basically it now involves the extensive use of tar products applied to the body as an ointment followed by total body ultraviolet light exposure in special ultraviolet B boxes. Ultraviolet-B light seems to potentiate the action of coal tar. In other words, the coal tar plus ultraviolet seem more effective when used together than when either is used alone.

A traditional Goeckerman program is mainly administered in the hospital or treatment center. This is necessary because of the staining properties of tar and prolonged nature of the treatment (two to four weeks for best results). There have been some recent changes.

First, more elegant, more cosmetic tar preparations have been developed. They are not as messy and are better suited for outpatient use.

Second, though six or seven daily treatments per week will be necessary to clear severe psoriasis, three to five daily treatments per week have been shown to be quite effective in patients with less severe psoriasis. The more frequent the treatments, the more rapidly the psoriasis will clear.

In some cases, lubricating cream and ointments can be substituted for tar in the Goeckerman program; however, more ultraviolet radiation is then necessary.

The Goeckerman treatment can be used for most types of psoriasis—mild to extensive. The outline of treatment is as follows:

1. The tar will be applied several hours before each light treatment.

2. The residual tar is wiped off, depending on which tar form is used. Tar oils, creams, and gels usually do not require removing before ultraviolet exposure.

3. Usually within two to four hours you will receive treatment in the ultraviolet cabinets.

4. The above procedures may be repeated later in the day.

What to Expect From the Goeckerman Program

In most patients clearing will begin in one to two weeks. This program produces *moderate* to *good* clearing after 12 to 20 treatments. Maximum clearing can be expected after 20 to 40 treatments. Some people clear faster. The general idea is to get you as clear as possible. The length of the program may depend on how many light treatments are taken weekly. Maintenance treatment at varying intervals helps to maintain clearance. If there is a relapse, the full program can be reinstated.

Anthralin Therapy

This has been previously mentioned. It may be combined with the Goeckerman program in selected patients to give a more rapid improvement of psoriasis.

Goeckerman and Anthralin at a Treatment Center or Hospital

The advantages of the Goeckerman and anthralin programs are their consistent benefits in most patients, long remission times (few months to sometimes greater than a year), and long-term safety.

If your psoriasis is very widespread or has failed to respond to the outpatient treatment, a period of treatment at the treatment center may be very beneficial. There are several benefits to such a visit.

First, you will get away from the stresses of your daily routine. This alone is quite beneficial. You will learn more about your psoriasis, as well as how to use the various medications. You will have a chance to talk to others with the same problems. Finally, you will undergo the Goeckerman and anthralin treatment for psoriasis.

What to Expect From the Treatment Center

Clearing proceeds over a two-to-four-week period. Remissions may last some months to over a year. Maintenance treatments can be continued in the office. With flare-ups, the Program can be reinstituted.

Photochemotherapy (Psoralen and Ultraviolet Light A): PUVA Program

This program is a combined drug and ultraviolet program. It is administered at a combined treatment center or as an outpatient program. With PUVA, psoralen (methoxsalen) is administered sometime before getting into a special ultraviolet-A light box. The light interacts with the psoralen and improves the psoriasis. Psoralen may also be administered by oral or topical routes.

This method is relatively new. It was first developed in 1974. It was approved by the FDA in 1982 but serious concerns still exist. There is concern about long-term side effects such as skin aging, skin cancer, damage to the immune system, eye changes, and effects on other body systems. Probably the full understanding of the side effects of PUVA will not be completely known until many years have gone by.

PUVA usually needs to be given three times weekly initially. As the psoriasis improves, less frequent treatments become possible.

What to Expect From the PUVA Treatment

You can expect improvement and, it is hoped, long-term control of your psoriasis.

Methotrexate

Methotrexate is a drug used to treat severe psoriasis. It is an FDA-approved internal medication used in the treatment of severe psoriasis.

When used properly, methotrexate has to be used carefully; when used improperly and without proper follow-up, it can be harmful, particularly to the liver. The decision as to whether you should take methotrexate will be made after you read the special information about this drug and have certain laboratory studies done. Most patients have to have liver biopsies performed before or at an early stage of therapy.

What to Expect From Treatment With Methotrexate

The average person will show some clearing in about four weeks. The number of doses to clear, the length of time you will stay clear, and the amount of methotrexate to maintain clearance will vary. Office visits are usually initially at one-week intervals and are gradually lengthened to usually once every four weeks.

Alternating and Combining of Programs

Sometimes you may move from one treatment to another, as your psoriasis changes. The aim is always to use the one that is best for you at that time. In addition, therapies may be combined.

PSORIASIS AND ARTHRITIS

About 10% of psoriasis patients have arthritis. If this occurs there are several oral medications (nonsteroid anti-inflammatory drugs—Indocin, Naprosyn, Motrin, Meclomen) that may help. The dermatologist may also decide to send the psoriasis patient to a rheumatologist specializing in joint disease.

RESEARCH TYPES OF TREATMENT

From time to time new drugs or modifications of available drugs are available for the treatment of some patients with different skin diseases. If such a treatment appears to be of potential help for your psoriasis then you may be offered a possible course of such a treatment.

Examples of current research treatments include alternative anthralins, alternative steroids, and alternative retinoids (all topical drugs), as well as new retinoids (e.g., etretinate, arotinoid ethylester), somatostatin (growth hormone), and alternative psoralens (all systemic drugs).

USEFUL ADDRESSES OF PSORIASIS ASSOCIATIONS FOR THE PSORIASIS PATIENT

United States
The National Psoriasis Foundation
Suite 200
415 SW Canyon Court
Portland, OR 97221
Britain
The Psoriasis Association
7 Milton Street
Northampton NN2 7JG
Canada
The Canadian Psoriasis Association
The Women's College Hospital
76 Greenville Street
Toronto, Ontario
Australia
The Skin and Psoriasis Foundation
PO Box 228
PO Collins Street
3000 Melbourne
New Zealand
The Auckland Psoriasis Society (Inc)
PO Box 3062
Auckland I

Index